When Love Hurts

A Woman's Guide to Understanding
Abuse in Relationships

Second Edition

When Love Hurts

A Woman's Guide to Understanding Abuse in Relationships

Jill Cory &
Karen McAndless-Davis

Second Edition

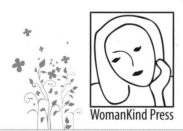

WomanKind Press

When Love Hurts : A Woman's Guide to Understanding Abuse in Relationships
Second Edition

Cover and page design by Pink Sheep Media
"Contemplative Woman" illustration by Carole Gignac
Editing by Emily Meetsma, Elizabeth Phinney (1st Ed.) and Jennifer Kingsley (2nd Ed.)

Printed in Canada on 100% post consumer recycled paper by:
Marquis Imprimeur
2700, rue Rachel est
Montréal, Québec H2H 1S7

Published by: WomanKind Press
                2313 Marine Drive
                New Westminster, BC, V3M 2H6
                www.womankind.bc.ca
                www.whenlovehurts.ca
                info@whenlovehurts.ca

10 9 8 7

Seventh Printing 2016

Library and Archives Canada Cataloguing in Publication

Cory, Jill, 1957-
   When love hurts : a woman's guide to understanding abuse in relationships / Jill Cory and Karen McAndless-Davis. -- 2nd ed.

ISBN 978-0-9686016-1-7

   1. Wife abuse. 2. Wife abuse--Prevention. 3. Women--Crimes against.
4. Women--Crimes against--Prevention. I. McAndless-Davis, Karen, 1965- II. Title.

HV6626.C66 2008   **362.82'92**   **C2007-907532-0**

Table of Contents

Chapter 9   Am I getting the support I need?

Chapter 10   Should I leave him?

Chapter 11   How do I heal from the abuse?

Afterword

Table of Exercises

Chapter 7   Why is my partner abusive?

Chapter 8   What's this doing to my kids?

Chapter 9   Am I getting the support I need?

Chapter 10   Should I leave him?

Chapter 11   How do I heal from the abuse?

Table of Diagrams

About the Authors

Jill Cory and Karen McAndless-Davis are friends and colleagues who share a deep compassion and respect for women who have experienced abuse. Together, they bring over three decades of experience to their work.

Jill began working with women in abusive relationships at the Calgary Women's Emergency Shelter in the early 1980s. After moving to Vancouver, she researched women's experiences in leaving abusive relationships. For the following seven years she developed and facilitated counseling programs for women and their abusive partners. Jill currently works at B.C. Women's Hospital and Health Centre supporting staff who respond to women experiencing abuse. Jill lives with David, her partner of 24 years, and their two children, Becky and Ben.

Karen's passion for this issue comes from personal experience. Her partner, Bruce, was abusive for the first ten years of their relationship. After several years of hard work (involving both group and individual counseling), Bruce changed his abusive behaviour and the beliefs underlying his actions. Karen and Bruce have now been happily married in a relationship of trust and respect for over ten years. They have two children, Luke and Isaac.

While Karen experienced abuse, she participated in a group counseling program. The support and encouragement that Karen received in this group kindled her desire to help other women living with abuse. For many years now, she has provided individual and group counseling to women in various communities. She also travels widely to provide training on the women-centered approach presented in "When Love Hurts."

Acknowledgments

We thank all of the women whom we have been privileged to know, support and learn from. Your desire for a safer future has taught us about the strength of the human spirit and our infinite capacity to care for each other. We would like to express our deep gratitude to you. Your wisdom and courage have inspired us to tell your stories.

We also want to thank the women who contributed to this book by giving us their invaluable insights and suggestions. Your comments and encouragement motivated and guided us.

Since the conception of this book, Bruce McAndless-Davis has been an amazing supporter. The first edition of this book would not have become a reality without his constant encouragement and hundreds of hours of work. He has worn many hats through our adventures in self-publishing, including publishing manager, bookkeeper and "tech guy." His dedication and support have been invaluable to us.

Special thanks to Pink Sheep Media for bringing their creativity, intelligence and ethics to the design of this edition.

Jill's acknowledgments: Karen, your wisdom and unwavering commitment to women's safety is a constant source of inspiration for me. What good fortune it has been for me to work and learn with you.

David, you have been my source of knowledge about respectful relationships between women and men. For that, I thank you deeply.

Karen's acknowledgments: Jill, your unfailing conviction that men and women can live in mutual, loving and respectful relationships inspired Bruce and me to live and love in a way that is truly a gift. Your belief that I had something to offer other women was the inspiration I needed to get started in this work. The deep respect and compassion with which you approach every woman is an attitude I feel grateful to have made my own.

Bruce, there have been many times in my work that have felt impossible. You have been a constant voice to say, "yes, you can!" Thank you.

Introduction

Love is meant to be supportive. We expect our partners to provide strength and comfort to us. But what happens when love hurts? What if your partner betrays your love by hurting you through his words or actions? You may feel confused, angry, sad or even depressed. It can be hard to know what to do or who to talk to. Perhaps you've told yourself, "My situation is not that bad" or "I'm exaggerating the problem." Maybe others have told you that your experiences are part of the normal ups and downs of a relationship. Maybe you think that the problem lies with you and you're the one who needs to change. You may have tried many times to make changes within your relationship, but you continue to be hurt.

You are not alone. In this book, you will meet other women who have been betrayed and hurt by their partners. You will hear these women describe the pain and confusion of their relationships and their journeys to find answers. We hope that their stories will help you to feel connected with others. We also hope that this book will help you to make sense of your own relationship.

About this book:

We wrote this book to make the material we use in our support groups available to as many women as possible. Over the years, we have seen how information about abuse is of great benefit to the women that we meet. We have included women's stories throughout this book for two purposes. The first is to help you, the reader, feel less alone. Many of the stories in this book will ring true for you. Up until now, you may have felt completely isolated in your situation. You are not. Second, we know that women learn from other women's experiences - drawing strength and insight from each other. We hope that, in hearing other women's stories, you will begin to hear your own story more clearly.

The exercises from our counseling program are also laid out in this book, and it is designed for you to write in. Recording your experiences can help you to clarify your thoughts. However, if you are still living with your partner, you may be concerned that he will find this book and use it against you. If this is a concern, you may decide not to include your personal thoughts. You may even want to hide the book entirely from your partner.

We encourage you to read this book at your own pace. Some women read this book quickly, feeling relieved to have finally found something that gives words to their experience. Other women read it slowly, wanting to absorb it bit by bit without being overwhelmed by the possible implications for their lives.

All of the stories in this book are true. Some of the stories are told of women; some of them are told by the women themselves. The names and identifying characteristics of all women have been changed to protect their privacy.

Why a second edition?

Since this book first came out, more than ten thousand copies have found their way into women's hands, and we have received a steady flow of enthusiastic appreciation from readers. At the same time, we know that many more women do not have enough information or support, and we wanted to make this book more widely available. We hope that this updated and expanded version will reach even more women, offering affirmation and hope.

Why the new chapter?

When we shared the first edition of this book with our focus groups, they told us that we needed a chapter about rebuilding and healing from abuse. That chapter was not in us at the time. At that point, we felt that each woman's journey to safety and wholeness was profoundly unique, and we didn't see the commonalities. Since that time, however, we have had the privilege of staying in touch with women for longer periods of time. Now that we have walked alongside women for years, common threads have emerged. The new chapter, like the rest of the book, is a reflection back to women of what we have learned from them.

Who is this book for?

First and foremost, this book is for women who have experienced abuse from their male partner. It addresses all forms of abuse including verbal, emotional, financial, sexual and physical. It was written to help make sense of a current or past relationship. We are not suggesting you stay in your relationship, and we are not suggesting you leave. Our goal is to provide you with information and support so that you can make your own decisions and gain greater control over your situation. If you are being hurt by the person you love, the fact that you love him may no longer be enough. It takes tremendous courage to begin to ask deeper questions. We trust that this book will help you find answers as you search for a brighter future.

Since this book was first published, we have discovered it also has a wider audience. Professionals supporting women who have experienced abuse will find this book helpful. Reading this book will assist you to better understand the complex situation women find themselves in. We encourage doctors, lawyers, religious leaders and others to keep a copy of this book available for their own reference and to loan to those seeking advice or direction. As well, many counselors, advocates, and shelter workers find this book a great guide for both individual and group counseling.

Similarly, friends and family will find this a helpful book. When someone we love is being hurt in a relationship, there is a natural impulse to stop the hurt as quickly as possible. Friends and family may make the mistake of oversimplifying the situation and pushing the woman to either leave the relationship or to "fix" it. Unfortunately, there is nothing simple about all the conflicting emotions and practical challenges of living with an abusive man. What women need most are support people who appreciate how difficult their situation is and can hang in with them during the long run. This book can help you to be that kind of person.

Jill Cory and Karen McAndless-Davis, Vancouver, BC. January 2008.

Allison's story

We begin our book with one woman's story. "Allison" is not this woman's real name, but her experiences are real. We hope that you will see aspects of your own life reflected in hers. At the same time, we know that every woman is unique, and parts of Allison's story will not be familiar to you. We also know that the choices Allison made may not be your choices. Every woman finds her own solutions; these are Allison's solutions, and this is her story.

I met Paul on an airplane flight. We struck up a conversation, and he said, "Why don't we get together for dinner and a movie?" meaning that we should move to the centre of the plane for the meal and film. It was unusual for men to pay attention to me, so when Paul did, I found it very flattering. I thought to myself, "Here's this handsome charming man talking to me. This is quite wonderful."

We talked for a long time on the plane, and I really enjoyed myself, but I also thought that after the flight we'd just go our separate ways. To my surprise, as the plane landed, he asked if we could get together the following evening. We went out for dinner and a play. That night I stayed over at his hotel, which was very romantic. It all seemed so exciting. Looking back, I realize that it happened so quickly I didn't have time to think it through.

We started dating. He called me all of the time and gave me small gifts and cards. No other man had ever treated me so nicely, and I felt swept off my feet. After a few months, I got a strange call from him in the middle of the night. He was drunk and pressuring me about something, and he just wouldn't let it go. This was my first indication that there was a problem. Still, it seemed to be an isolated event; I didn't want to make a big deal out of it.

We did lots of fun things together, but I always had an anxious feeling in the pit of my stomach. When I expressed doubts about the relationship, Paul reassured me by saying, "Don't worry, my job is to win you over."

Paul put a lot of pressure on me to live with him, and he also asked me to marry him early on. It was very confusing—he seemed so committed, but at the same time I didn't like feeling pressured to move things along quickly. He said he wanted to have children with me. This appealed to me as I was 29, I really wanted kids, and it seemed to be the right time in my life for a family.

While we were dating, things seemed to be working out, but I often felt frustrated. Paul never quite understood me; even when I explained things very carefully, he would misinterpret me. He would get angry and insist I had said things I knew I hadn't. This would make me question my competence, my sanity. I put so much effort into communicating, and he never did. It was exhausting.

One night while I was driving us to a friend's party, we began arguing, and he hit me on the leg. I stopped the car, and he started screaming. I was really frightened. At other times during our relationship he would slap or hit me, and sometimes I would hit back. No one had ever hit me before, and I had certainly never hit anyone either.

I became clinically depressed and went to see my doctor about antidepressants. My doctor asked, "Are you sure you aren't just depressed about your relationship?" I said my relationship was good, but looking back on it I see that a lot of my depression was related to Paul.

Around this time, Paul and I also started to see a counselor. When I revealed that Paul had hit me, the counselor said he wouldn't work with couples if there was any violence. He told me that I had to stop pushing Paul's buttons and that Paul had to stop hitting me. (Paul still refers to this counselor's advice many years later by suggesting that our relationship problems were all about me "pushing his buttons.") Because the counselor was a professional, I wanted to take his advice even though it didn't feel right to me.

I wanted to buy a place of my own, but we just sort of ended up looking for a place to live in together. I had doubts about buying a home with Paul, but the day the deal went through, I found out I was pregnant. Getting pregnant wasn't unexpected, and we were both pleased. It became very hard to say no to all of this—a new home, a baby, a partner. I figured I just hadn't pushed myself hard enough in other relationships. I thought, "These are my insecurities, and I just need to work through this."

Once we got into our own place, the fights escalated. One night during a disagreement, Paul started smashing a crystal tumbler against my head repeatedly. It was the first time he'd really hurt me. I probably needed stitches, but I didn't go to the hospital. I was fifteen weeks pregnant and felt emotionally and physically vulnerable. I didn't tell anyone because

I knew others would want me to leave, and I knew I wasn't going to. Now that I was pregnant, I thought, "I need to make this work."

When Alex was born, Paul was more supportive during labour than I'd ever hoped, but the next night he called me at the hospital very late. He screamed at me for talking so much to the midwife during the delivery and "flirting" with the doctor. His ranting was awful, but at the same time he did some very nice things, and I was very confused.

Once we got home with the baby, it was all up to me. Paul never dressed, bathed, fed, or changed Alex. I had just assumed that Paul and I were in this together and was disappointed at his self-centredness.

Even at this point, we still had lots of fun together, but it was always interspersed with bad times. We liked to go out to nice restaurants, but there was always tension because I never knew what would set him off.

I finally got some information about a support group for women who have been abused. At first I was hesitant, but hearing other women's stories was so powerful. I immediately felt that this was a group of women who understood me and all of the crazy stuff that was going on with Paul.

Paul was less physically abusive after the baby was born, but he was much more emotionally and financially abusive. This was confusing because, in some ways, it seemed that things were better, but I actually felt more controlled and intimidated. I see now that Paul just got smarter about his abuse. He appeared to be managing his anger by not hitting me, but he used his anger to be abusive in other ways. It was hard for me to consider leaving when I didn't feel physically at risk. It has taken a long time for me to figure out what's normal arguing and what's abuse.

Because I could be nasty sometimes, I thought I was at fault. I often felt that Paul's abuse was justified. Sometimes I would blame myself because I felt I had started things. I thought these were arguments, but they were really about Paul staying in control.

A lot of things kept me from leaving the relationship. I thought I was a failure if I couldn't make it work, and I really wanted a family for Alex and me. I loved my little home and didn't want to leave it, and anytime I suggested I might leave, Paul threatened me. He also told me that he would want joint custody, and I really didn't want that for Alex.

We did eventually separate, but Paul made that very difficult too. He fought me on custody, access and support payments.

Once I got some distance from Paul, his abuse continued, but it didn't affect me nearly as much. The ongoing support of my women's group, family and friends was crucial.

Some of the decisions that I had to make were really hard, and I never had any guarantees that things would work out. But our lives are so much better and happier now, despite Paul's ongoing attempts to undermine and control us. Alex and I are happy in our own little home and neighbourhood; the two of us are a family. Not all women need to leave their relationship to feel safe, but I did.

1

Am I experiencing abuse?

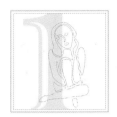

I didn't see myself as an abused woman. The only images I had came from television. I thought of abused women as weak, quiet and less educated—women who were battered and bruised. That wasn't who I was at all. And my partner certainly didn't fit my image of an abusive husband. I thought they were wild and out of control—men who drank too much, were brutal and hateful. My partner's behaviour was confusing. I saw him being kind and pleasant to our friends and family. He was often loving to me, and I loved him. But he got angry so easily; and when he was angry, he was hurtful. Since his hurtful behaviour was always directed at me, I believed I was the cause of the abuse. **Maggie**

Am I an "abused woman"?

Was it difficult for you to pick up this book? Is it hard even to consider if you are being abused in your relationship? If it is a struggle even to ask the question, you are not alone. Many women find it hard to imagine that they are being abused by their partners. Part of the struggle has to do with the negative stereotype our culture has of "battered women" and "abusive men." If neither you nor your partner fit the stereotype, it may be even harder to imagine that you're actually being abused.

Women who are abused by their partners are like any other women. Some are professionals, some are homemakers, some are wealthy, some are poor. Women who experience abuse come from all racial and ethnic backgrounds. In the same way, abusive men don't fit the stereotype either. The stereotype is of men who are monstrous and volatile. It does not reflect that these men are often affectionate, charming and sociable. Some men even appear to be progressive in their attitudes about women.

The stereotype of an "abused woman" may prevent women from being able to describe or identify their experience. You may have struggled between your experience of abuse and the negative stereotype of an "abused woman." We encourage you to pay attention to your experience rather than to the stereotype.

It might be useful for you to identify all the negative descriptions associated with the stereotype. Take a moment to think about the stereotypes many people hold about abused or "battered" women. Jot down the stereotypes you or others hold.

Would you define yourself in terms of these stereotypes? Of course not. None of us would. Thankfully, not one of them is true. There is only one thing that women who are experiencing abuse have in common: they are being abused by their partners. It sounds straightforward, doesn't it? But it's amazing how many ideas distract us from this basic truth.

You will notice as you read this book that we always refer to "women who experience abuse," and not "abused" or "battered women." That is because women are much more than the abuse they experience. You are a person with many qualities and gifts. There is nothing typical about a woman experiencing abuse, except for the abuse itself.

Many women feel that, because they do not fit the stereotype, they are not being abused. Abuse takes many forms and, even though you don't fit the stereotype, you may well be experiencing emotional, physical, financial or sexual abuse from your partner. You may even have been asking yourself if your partner is abusive. This book will help you to know if you are being abused. If you have picked up this book, you are obviously not comfortable with the dynamics in your relationship or with your partner's behaviour.

As I started to read about abuse and attend my support group for women I had very conflicting emotions. On the one hand, it was good to finally figure out what was really going on in my relationship. On the other hand, I struggled with feeling ashamed that somehow this had happened to me. I was also scared that if I really admitted that I was being abused, I would then have to leave my partner. That was something I really didn't want to do. Looking back on it now, I realize that those conflicting emotions were only natural and all I could do was be patient and gentle with myself. **Sarah**

What's wrong in my relationship?

You may have asked yourself, "What's wrong in my relationship?" You have probably considered many explanations in order to try to understand the problem. Let's look at some of these explanations.

Most ideas about relationship problems suggest that men and women are equally responsible. Sayings such as "It takes two to tango" reflect this cultural belief. In relationships that are respectful, and when women are not worried about how their partners will respond or behave, we agree that men and women share responsibility for problems in the relationship. There is a problem with the idea of shared responsibility, however, when a man is controlling or abusive. In such cases it is often assumed that the woman has done something to cause the abuse—she has provoked him. In one way or another, women are often held partially responsible for the abuse in their relationship.

In our experience, women who are being abused seek many solutions and explanations in order to improve their relationship. You may have gone to counseling by yourself or with your partner, or you may have asked your partner to attend an anger management program (or attended one yourself). Perhaps you have read other self-help books that have suggested that the problem has to do with the natural differences between men and women and that you simply need to accept your partner the way he is. Other books may have implied that you are codependent, love too much, or have problems asserting yourself. Based on suggestions from counselors or self-help books, you have probably tried to change your behaviour in order to get your partner to treat you with respect.

If you are experiencing abuse, the problem will persist no matter what you try to change about yourself, your partner or your relationship. This is because the problem is his abuse—his need to have control in your relationship. The sad truth is that you can't change the one thing that really matters—stopping your partner's abuse. Only he can choose to stop being abusive. Until then, everything that takes place in the relationship is related to the abuse. When a man is abusive in his relationship, he alone is responsible for the abuse, but there are things you can do for yourself. This book will help you to understand your situation and it will suggest ways to care for yourself and your children.

Why was I attracted to him?

Remember when you first met your partner? Did he act in the same abusive ways he does now? When he first met you, did he shake your hand and say, "Hello, my name is Bob and I am abusive. Let's move in together"? Of course not. If he had, you wouldn't have had anything more to do with him! Similarly, if on your first date he'd treated you the way he treats you now, would you have had a second date?

In reflecting back on their relationship, women describe the early period as generally being positive and loving. They didn't observe any abusive behaviour until they were committed to the relationship. When women in group counseling list the positive qualities they saw in their partner when they first met him, they always generate a substantial list. Like you, none of these women thought abuse could happen to them.

Sometimes women describe their partner as a hardworking and stable man. Sometimes their partner appears to be a "good family man" in that he seems to be good with children or to value family connections. Sometimes women will reflect on how thoughtful their partner was or that they found their partner easy to talk with or fun to be around.

You may describe different things that attracted you to your partner. Whatever they were, they were positive qualities. Think back to your first experiences of your partner and all the things that you were attracted to in him. What interested you about him? Remember, you are making a list of the qualities you saw in him when you first met him, not those you see in him now.

Look over the characteristics you thought your partner had. Don't they seem to be attractive and positive? It's important to remind yourself that you were attracted to good things in your partner. You were not attracted to the abuse. The list you've made above is a list that anyone, in any relationship, could generate about their partner.

When you first began your relationship, much in it seemed positive to you. If that hadn't been the case, you probably would have ended the relationship before it really began. And, of course, your partner still has some good qualities. [1]

How did I get here?

When you first met your partner, you probably experienced a period of courtship that was enjoyable and that firmly established your relationship. At some point while dating him, however, something may have happened that made you uncomfortable. Perhaps your partner raised his voice, accused you of having an affair, swore at you, argued relentlessly or threw something.

For some women, the first experience of abuse can be even more subtle. For example, perhaps he was very late for a date and didn't offer an appropriate apology or explanation. Or maybe your partner told mutual friends a private and embarrassing story about you. Remind yourself, however, that regardless of what your partner's first disrespectful or abusive behaviour was, it happened within the context of lots of positive things.

You probably overlooked that first instance of bad behaviour. You had some good reasons for overlooking it. Your partner probably offered explanations for his behaviour or may have apologized to you. Because you are a generous person, you probably accepted his explanation or apology. Perhaps you reminded yourself that no one is perfect and that it is normal for couples to disagree. You may also have reminded yourself of all the good qualities in your partner—the things you appreciated about him. So, after some discomfort over his behaviour, you tried to let the incident go so that you could feel connected and close to your partner.

If your partner's poor behaviour had been a one-time incident, there would be no problem. But there was a next time and a next time and a next time.

What can I do?

Our goal in writing this book is to offer you an opportunity to make sense of your relationship for yourself. We have noticed that many women who have been subjected to their partners' opinions and interpretations do not feel safe in expressing their own ideas. As you read through this book, we hope that you will be able to interpret your

---

1 Note: Sometimes women are abused in more than one of their intimate relationships. If this is true for you, simply evaluate one relationship at a time as you work through this book.

relationship and your partner's behaviour in a way that reflects your own experiences, thoughts, feelings and insights. Through this process you can describe for yourself who you are, what you expect and what you need from your partner.

You are probably already doing many things to make sense of your situation—meeting your needs and planning your immediate and long-term future. Perhaps you don't realize or appreciate all the mental and emotional work this entails. Reading this book and other books, getting appropriate counseling, resting during a lull in the relationship, making lists, putting money aside, trying to nurture your children and keep them safe—these are all examples of actively looking after yourself. Remember that each of these small steps is extremely important!

Something else you can do at this time is to observe your partner's behaviour and compare this with the promises your partner has made to you. We call this work evidence gathering. It means looking at your partner's behaviour as the clearest sign of his intentions. It is giving his actions more weight than his words. For example, if your partner promises to be more truthful with you but continues to lie, you might begin to wonder if what he does is more meaningful than what he says.

While women find the concept of evidence gathering helpful, many also struggle with having to gather evidence about their partner. For some women, it feels wrong to assess their partner's behaviour in this way. However, women so often tell us that their partner doesn't fulfill his promises, the very promises that have kept them hopeful and encouraged about the possibility of change in their relationship. We therefore think that focusing on the evidence of his behaviour rather than on his promises can help to clarify what's going on in your relationship and help you feel less confused. We hope that the information you gather will help you make the best plans for any future action.

In the next chapter, we will explore some of the evidence in your relationship so that you can begin to understand what is happening for you.

2

What is the Cycle of Abuse?

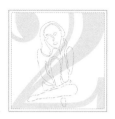

> My partner's behaviour was so crazy making. It seemed random and out of control. He would blow up over the smallest things. Looking at the Cycle of Abuse helped me start to make sense of my partner's behaviour; it had a pattern and a purpose.   *Sheila*

Is there a pattern?

Most women, living with an abusive partner, find it hard to see any pattern to the abuse. His behaviour seems bizarre and unpredictable. It seems unbelievable that the same person, who is kind and affectionate one day, could be cruel and malicious another. His hurtful behaviour seems to come as isolated events. You may think of him as a generally "good guy" who does some really awful things once in a while.

When we share with women the belief that abuse does have a pattern, they begin to see it for themselves. This pattern of behaviour is called the Cycle of Abuse.[1] There are three distinct phases to the Cycle. Each of the phases is abusive, but in different ways and with different effects on you. We will review each phase, first by describing your partner's behaviour.

The three phases of the Cycle of Abuse are called honeymoon, tension-building and explosion.

The Cycle begins with the honeymoon, which women often describe as an intense period of courtship. During this time, the relationship first gets established. We've described the first occurrence of the honeymoon in chapter 1. Your partner's behaviour during

---

1 Lenore E. Walker, *The Battered Woman* (New York: Harper and Row, Publishers, 1979), pp.55ff.

Diagram 2.1   The Cycle of Abuse

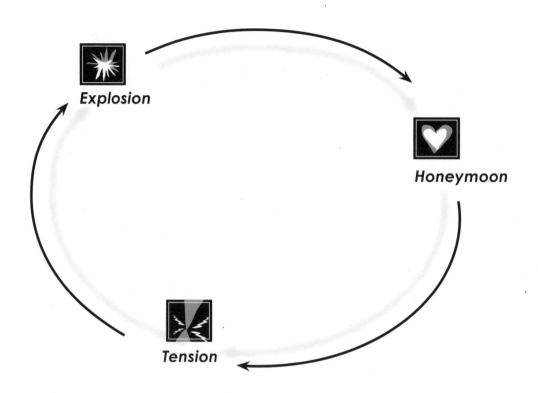

the honeymoon period seems positive. He is attentive and considerate. He may give you gifts or make promises, or he may simply behave in a way that seems acceptable or "normal." The two of you begin to establish a relationship together.

Then comes a period of tension-building. This phase of the Cycle will vary in length. Some abusive men may be sullen, silent, unpredictable or moody for a period of minutes, hours, weeks or months, creating unbearable tension in the relationship. The man's behaviour during this time may be angry or hostile. Women often describe their partners as being very critical of them. Some men withdraw from the relationship and appear disinterested and distant. They may justify this behaviour with excuses such as stress from work or financial concerns. They may also explain their behaviour by blaming their partners or children for creating the problems. Men will often deny that there is a problem, insisting that there is nothing wrong with their behaviour. Sometimes women feel that they are walking on eggshells, living in fear and trying to avoid the next explosion.

The final phase of the Cycle is the explosion. The first time you experienced an explosion, it may not have seemed that significant, but it probably distressed you. Perhaps your partner raised his voice at you or swore at you. Perhaps he slammed a door or banged down a pot. Perhaps he walked away and gave you the "silent treatment." If the Cycle has continued for years, the explosion phase becomes marked by increasingly brutal attacks, whether they are physical, verbal, psychological or sexual. The attacks also occur more frequently than at the beginning of the relationship.

After the explosion, your partner probably returns to the honeymoon phase. He stops the negative behaviour he demonstrated during the tension-building and explosion phases and behaves again in a seemingly positive way. Your partner may apologize and promise not to act in such a manner again, or he may simply resume behaving in a way that is acceptable to you. There are many tactics that he may use to convince you to stay with him. Being a caring, forgiving person, you accept his apology or reformed behaviour, and your relationship, and the Cycle, continue.

You may notice over time that your partner's behaviour during the tension-building and explosion phases becomes more extreme. His behaviour during the honeymoon phase may also change; he may give more gifts and make more promises in order to "win you back." Alternatively, some women find that the honeymoon period virtually disappears, and the relationship becomes characterized by the tension-building and explosion phases.

Diagram 2.2   The Cycle of Abuse: Examples of His Behaviour

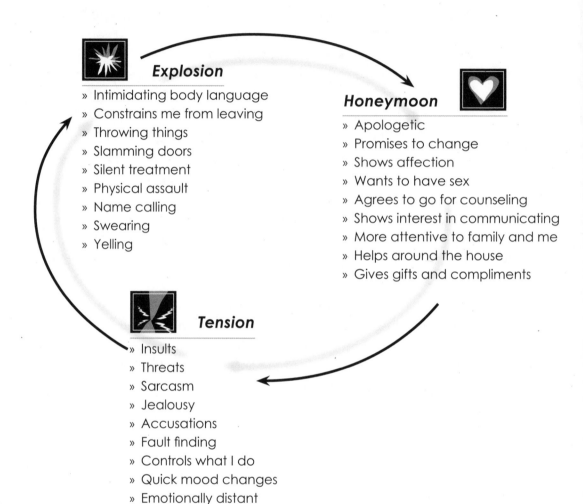

Explosion

- » Intimidating body language
- » Constrains me from leaving
- » Throwing things
- » Slamming doors
- » Silent treatment
- » Physical assault
- » Name calling
- » Swearing
- » Yelling

Honeymoon

- » Apologetic
- » Promises to change
- » Shows affection
- » Wants to have sex
- » Agrees to go for counseling
- » Shows interest in communicating
- » More attentive to family and me
- » Helps around the house
- » Gives gifts and compliments

Tension

- » Insults
- » Threats
- » Sarcasm
- » Jealousy
- » Accusations
- » Fault finding
- » Controls what I do
- » Quick mood changes
- » Emotionally distant

Above is a diagram of the Cycle of Abuse, drawn by a group of women who live with abusive men. It will give you some examples of the behaviour that abusive men demonstrate during each of these phases.

The Cycle of Abuse: My Experience of His Behaviour

(diagram showing the cycle)

Explosion → **Honeymoon** → **Tension** → (back to Explosion)

Perhaps you would now like to complete a Cycle for yourself. Beginning with the honeymoon phase, describe the seemingly appropriate behaviour that your partner demonstrates. Then list the behaviour your partner demonstrates during the tension-building phase and, finally, the explosion phase.

Women tell us that trying to manage the relationship and avoid the tension-building and explosion phases consumes all of their energy and concentration. There is little time to reflect on these patterns. We hope that drawing a Cycle for yourself has provided you with an opportunity to identify the pattern in your relationship.

When is a honeymoon not a honeymoon?

For many women, the honeymoon phase is the most confusing part of the Cycle. Your partner behaves in ways that appear to be loving or remorseful, but you may still feel uncomfortable. This confusion may keep you in your relationship. It is often when a woman feels ready to "give up on the relationship," possibly even making plans to move out, that her partner changes his behaviour or at least promises to do so; she then finds herself re-engaged in the relationship. During the honeymoon phase, your partner appears to be kind to you, but it is a manipulative type of kindness. Let's look at an example.

Irene

Irene has been unhappy in her marriage for a long time. She has considered leaving her partner on several occasions. One night, she and Dean argued for several hours about their financial situation. Dean kept escalating the argument until he was screaming at her and calling her names. Dean's behaviour frightened Irene, and she resolved to move out. The next morning, Dean helped to get the children off to school (something he never did) and apologized very sincerely for his behaviour the previous evening. He admitted that he had a problem with his anger and promised to take an anger management course. Irene is encouraged by his help with the children, his sincere apology, and his promise to seek counseling. She decides to give the relationship one more chance.

The honeymoon phase keeps you working on the relationship. If the relationship consisted only of tension-building and explosion, you may have left a long time ago. However, your partner is not always explosive; sometimes his behaviour seems acceptable and you feel attracted to him. Your partner seems sincere in what he says during the honeymoon phase, and you want to believe him. Because his behaviour during the honeymoon phase seems positive and because you hope that this time the change will be genuine and permanent, you stay in the relationship. For this reason, some women describe the honeymoon as a period of entrapment—the hope your partner raises is the hook keeping you involved. It is certainly not a honeymoon in the usual sense of the word.

The honeymoon phase is confusing because what appears to be caring behaviour is often controlling. You may find this idea difficult. Let's explore it further. Think about some of the things your partner offers during the honeymoon phase, such as a gift, a promise, an apology, sex. How do you feel about accepting what he has offered? Although you may feel grateful that the explosion is over, do you sometimes feel unready to accept the peace offering?

Women often feel unable to refuse what is being offered (or forced on them) during the honeymoon phase. They know there will be negative consequences if they decline the offer. When you understand this dynamic, you can understand that your partner's gestures during the honeymoon phase are still largely about controlling you. Your partner may appear to be genuinely concerned for you. However, his actions are still about staying in control.

Let's think this through in more concrete terms. Are you free to reject his overtures during the honeymoon time without fear of abuse? (We don't suggest you actually do this because it might be dangerous for you. Simply ask yourself if you could.) For example, if he comes home during a honeymoon phase with an expensive gift, are you free not to accept it? Although you may wish he had not spent money on jewellery when there are bills to pay, are you free to say so? If he suggests going on a walk together, are you free to say "no"? Can you tell him you are too tired for a walk without eventual negative consequences?

Imagine this scenario: You and a friend are hosting a dinner party together. After you have arranged to use her house because it is larger, you find out that she's been sick all week. Wanting to help her, you offer to do some of her house cleaning. Being embarrassed by the state of her house, your friend kindly declines your offer. How do you respond? Can you imagine responding with abuse? Can you imagine telling your friend that she's stupid for not accepting your offer, that she is going to ruin your party and that you are so insulted you will no longer attend? Of course you wouldn't respond this way, but this may be the way your partner behaves when you don't respond the way he wants during the honeymoon phase.

If you do not feel free to decline your partner's overtures during the honeymoon phase, it says something quite painful about his motives. If something is offered as a "gift" or "kind gesture," you should feel free to accept it or not. If your partner doesn't give you that choice, clearly he is focusing on his need to stay in control rather than on your well-being. If you don't go along with the honeymoon, he may become abusive. Some abusive men also become sulky or accuse their partners of being "unwilling to work on the relationship."

Your partner's overtures during the honeymoon stage certainly look sincere, but over time you begin to experience them differently. He is behaving as he does in order to have things his way, not out of a real interest in caring for you or in nurturing the relationship. His "kindness" is actually very manipulative. This may be a painful realization for you. It can be devastating to recognize that the honeymoon phase is also about your partner controlling you. An example from one woman's story helps to illustrate this point.

Janine

Janine was given a cell phone as a gift during a honeymoon phase. She didn't want the phone but was unable to decline the gift. Now her partner has even greater control over her. She can no longer even go to the grocery store without fear of him calling to ask what she's doing. "For her safety" he insists that she carry it with her always. If she leaves it behind, she is told she is forgetful and doesn't appreciate his gift.

The honeymoon phase leaves women feeling confused precisely because it is confusing. Some aspects of the honeymoon keep you feeling hopeful while at other times you simply feel trapped. Some women choose to leave during the honeymoon; it may feel like a safer time to do so. Other women, while wanting to leave, feel guilty about leaving. Their partner has made promises of change, and they feel obligated to stick around and "give him one more chance."

Who is in control of the Cycle?

The Cycle of Abuse is your partner's cycle. He is in control of it. Through it, he uses a variety of tactics to achieve his goal of maintaining power over you. You may not have thought of his behaviour in this way before—perhaps it has always seemed random to you. Maybe you've described his behaviour as out of control rather than a means of maintaining control.

Some women believe that they are responsible for the Cycle or that they cause the abuse. Your partner may even have suggested this. He will tell you that he lost his temper only because you were "pushing his buttons." Women may also feel that they are driving the Cycle because some of their own behaviour looks explosive or controlling.

Sometimes there is a period of escalation before the explosion. It is not uncommon for a woman to yell, swear, throw something or even hit her partner during this very tense period. In our experience, women behaving in this way are most often attempting to defend themselves. Women may sometimes behave in ways that seem explosive in an attempt to end the tension-building phase. If your partner has been increasing the tension for days or is building it to a level that is no longer tolerable for you, you may do something to break the tension-building phase and move into the inevitable explosion. You may or may not be aware of doing this.

> I remember thinking that my partner seemed determined to pick a fight, so we might as well get it over with. I would then stand up for myself in a given argument, and the explosion would inevitably come. During the first several years of our marriage, I occasionally yelled, swore or threw something at my partner. Once, after three hours of unrelenting emotional attacks, I slammed down an iron and broke it. All of this behaviour concerned me. It was not the way I wanted to be in my relationship. Now that my partner is no longer abusive, I no longer do the things that disturbed me. *Sandi*

Although you may have behaved in ways that are unacceptable to you, it is important to emphasize that your partner is the one who controls the Cycle of Abuse. The explosion will inevitably come. No matter what you do, your partner will find some reason to be abusive. He will attempt to use your behaviour to justify his explosion, but it does not. He will equate your "bad" behaviour with his, but they are not equal. Your motives are not the same. He is attempting to regain control and is using abusive tactics to do that. You are attempting to protect your physical and mental well-being and attempting to be heard or to have some say in your relationship.

Is the Cycle the same for everyone?

Hopefully you are connecting on some level with our description of the Cycle of Abuse. For some women it rings true the first time they encounter it. Other women need to explore the Cycle a bit and perhaps even modify it to better reflect their experiences. The Cycle may not be as tidy and predictable in real life as it is typed out on a piece of paper. It may not move predictably from one phase to the other. The phases may blur together, and they may not follow each other in order. Your partner may jump from phase to phase or linger a long time in one of them.

> For myself, I needed to put the emphasis on the different kinds of behaviour my partner demonstrated rather than on the Cycle itself. I wasn't aware so much of us moving in a Cycle as I was of my partner demonstrating three different kinds of behaviour. He certainly demonstrated honeymoon behaviour, tension-building behaviour and explosion behaviour. Sometimes, however, he moved the Cycle directly from honeymoon to explosion, and sometimes he moved it from explosion back to tension-building without a

honeymoon period. For these reasons, I found it helpful to draw out a Cycle of Abuse that described my own experience.

I imagined the Cycle as a combination padlock, because it illustrated clearly who was at the centre of the Cycle and who was controlling it. My partner was the dial on the padlock. He was in the centre and the controlling force of the Cycle. He chose where we would be on the Cycle and what behaviour he would use to achieve his goal of staying in control. The padlock also helped me to realize that the Cycle wouldn't necessarily move from honeymoon to tension-building to explosion; it might jump backwards or skip a phase. *Emma*

We hope you will take what you've read in this chapter and continue to think about it as you reflect on your partner's current or past behaviour. It can take some time to really see how the Cycle of Abuse is played out in your relationship, but understanding the pattern of abuse is helpful. For example, being able to anticipate the stages of the Cycle may allow you to plan for your safety during the explosion phase.

Understanding the Cycle in its entirety helps you to see what a difficult situation you are in. It is like living with Dr. Jekyll and Mr. Hyde. Each phase of the Cycle is a different expression of abuse, and you are left constantly trying to anticipate what is coming next. The honeymoon phase is often the most confusing because you see the man you were first attracted to and it rekindles hope in you. The tension-building phase of the Cycle of Abuse is different. There is a constant fear that, at any time, your partner could become explosive. Living with the anticipation of abuse is extremely exhausting and frightening. We say this not to make you feel hopeless but to help you recognize the tremendous strain under which you live.

In the next chapter, we will focus on your experiences during the Cycle of Abuse. This focus may help you appreciate more fully the complex and difficult situation you are in.

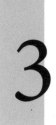

3

How do I experience the Cycle of Abuse?

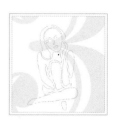

In subtle ways he tried to control my actions and my thoughts. He always had to prove that he was right and that I was wrong; we couldn't simply disagree. His rage would silence me. I constantly had to decide whether an issue was worth raising with him—if it was safe to bring it up. If he did any housework, he became angry and resentful. He was always picking fights and it was hard to avoid explosive situations. I was exhausted living with him. As time went on, John seemed angry more and more. Finally, when John broke my rib I began to see the seriousness of our situation. I wondered if this was abuse.
Lorena

Why do I feel so confused?

In this chapter, we look at the Cycle of Abuse as you experience it. Looking at the Cycle as a whole is important in order to understand how the abuse has really affected you. Throughout the Cycle you experience many different reactions and emotions in response to your partner's behaviours. Some of the reactions seem quite contradictory to each other. You may find yourself feeling love and hate, anger and affection, fear and intimacy. It is distressing to live with such a range of emotional reactions.

As well as leaving you exhausted and off-balance, your partner's constantly changing behaviour also has an effect on your self-identity. All of us count on the people around us to reflect a realistic picture of who we are. With your partner, you are getting a distorted picture that is constantly changing—and often very damaging. If during the explosion phase you are told that you are stupid and ugly but then during the honeymoon phase you are told you are attractive and fun to be around, it is difficult to get a very true picture of yourself and hold on to it.

While your partner is at the centre of it and controls it, the Cycle has a profound effect on you. Let's reflect on your experience of each phase of the Cycle.

Why does the honeymoon phase make me feel crazy?

As you may have already concluded from the previous chapter, the honeymoon phase can be the most difficult phase to figure out. Women can have different kinds of reactions which, at first glance, may seem rather distinct from each other.

Women are often most hopeful during the honeymoon phase, especially early in their relationship. Being hopeful makes a lot of sense. Your partner is doing something positive. Maybe he's apologized for his explosive behaviour; or he's promised never to behave that way again; or he's being considerate (e.g., encouraging you to spend more time with friends); or he's agreed to go for counseling. During this phase of the Cycle, you may do enjoyable things together (e.g., enjoy conversation, have sex, go on family outings). This may be a time when you can relax and recover from the explosion. These positive experiences may make you feel reconnected to your partner and encourage you to think that your relationship is on the mend. This makes sense—your partner's behaviour during this phase is intended to create hope in you so that you will stay in the relationship.

Some women, after experiencing the Cycle—perhaps hundreds of times—begin to question the sincerity of the honeymoon phase. If your partner apologizes for swearing at you and then does so in the very next argument, you will begin to doubt the genuineness of his apology. Similarly, if he promises to go for counseling but never manages to make an appointment, you may begin to doubt his promises. Based on this evidence, you may begin to feel skeptical during the honeymoon phase. Women sometimes feel guilty that they don't trust their partner's intentions during the honeymoon phase. We think this skepticism reflects your wisdom. Your experience gives you plenty of evidence to wonder whether he will keep his promises. While you still might be hopeful, you are also allowing yourself to pay attention to the evidence he is presenting to you. It may be very painful for you to be skeptical about someone you love.

As we discussed in chapter 2, the honeymoon phase can also feel entrapping for women. The honeymoon phase keeps you committed to the relationship. It also serves to control you. You may not feel free to reject your partner's overtures during the honeymoon phase. You might feel coerced into going along with him, even if you disagree. For example, if your partner wants to have sex during this phase, you may not feel free to say "no." If you do, he may become angry or sulky, or he may also accuse you of being cold and distant.

Many women express fear of doing or saying anything that will "set off" their partners and ruin the relative peace of the honeymoon phase. Feeling forced to go along with the honeymoon wears on a woman's self-esteem. Women feel that they are not being true to themselves as they are pressured to go along with their partner's ideas of what is needed to set things right.

Given the myriad of emotions that are invoked, it makes sense for you to have a range of reactions during the honeymoon phase. It makes sense to feel hopeful, skeptical, trapped, or fearful. Your partner is doing things that can make you feel any or all of these things. It also makes sense if some days you feel skeptical and some days you feel hopeful and some days you feel trapped. The honeymoon phase is really crazy-making!

Below is a list of things women have experienced during the honeymoon phase of the Cycle. See if some of these experiences seem familiar to you.

During the Honeymoon Phase, I...

☐ feel like things are going well

☐ feel safe and secure

☐ feel generous

☐ feel loved and appreciated

☐ feel relaxed

☐ can ask for things

☐ feel like I can express myself

☐ think the relationship is not so bad

☐ feel hopeful

☐ feel positive

☐ feel grateful

☐ enjoy my partner's attention

☐ feel loving and want to be intimate

☐ feel sorry for him

☐ feel energetic

☐ feel free to see friends

☐ feel safe to ask him to do stuff

☐ feel like I should try harder

☐ feel guilty

☐ feel confused

☐ feel skeptical

☐ become introspective

☐ question the relationship

☐ know he is not being genuine

☐ wonder how long it will last

☐ feel doubtful

☐ feel uncomfortable

☐ feel fake

☐ feel dead/numb

☐ feel distant

☐ feel repelled by his approaches

☐ want to escape

☐ _____

☐ _____

☐ _____

☐ _____

The honeymoon phase tends to be a time of conflicting emotions and thoughts, leaving you uncertain and confused.

Why do I feel like I'm walking on eggshells?

Now ask yourself what happens to you during the tension phase of the Cycle? Many women feel they are "walking on eggshells." Your partner seems angry, hostile or stressed out. For your safety, you do whatever you can to keep things from getting worse. You may try to be very accommodating during this phase, making everything in the home positive and calm. If you have children, you may have learned to keep them quiet or out of sight. You may attempt to respond to all your partner's requests or demands, but no matter what you do, he continues to be demanding, critical or sullen.

During this tension phase, you may also begin to feel frustrated. It may feel that no matter what you do, he maintains a high level of tension. He may keep trying to pick fights. Perhaps you feel that he is hyper-critical of everything you do—it feels as if you can't do anything without his judgment.

The crazy-making part of the tension phase is that your partner will constantly change the rules. For example, maybe he gets angry when you disagree with him about something. In the hopes of trying to keep things calm, you decide to keep your opinions to yourself. Then he tells you that you are infuriating him because you will not speak your mind. Changing the rules keeps your partner in charge and keeps you desperately trying to figure out how to behave, what to say, what to wear and even where to look. You may find yourself always second-guessing your own decisions. For example, the first time you wore a new dress he told you how beautiful you looked, but the next time you wore that dress he accused you of looking like a whore and having an affair. So how do you decide whether or not to wear that dress again? Women who have experienced abuse describe an endless number of examples similar to this, saying that there is no way to anticipate their partner's response or make a decision that will keep them safe. They feel that they can't do anything right and live in constant fear of taking a step that will lead to the next explosion.

Often women notice physical problems as a result of living with the fear and uncertainty. The extreme stress you are under may lead to health concerns such as headaches, heart palpitations, dizziness, exhaustion or insomnia. Some women also feel depressed or anxious during this period of the Cycle. Here's how one woman described her experience:

> I would make sure the house was in perfect order before my husband came home from work. This was always a challenge because I ran a daycare out of my home. No matter how hard I worked to make everything look nice, he would always find something to get angry about. I began to be scared day after day, dreading his arrival home from work. I felt very emotional. My blood pressure went up. The kids began to pick up on my fear. I doubted myself and blamed myself. I kept wondering what I could do to change the situation. I now understand it was not me who had to change. *Jane*

To reflect on what is happening for you during this phase of the Cycle, it might be helpful to think of one situation in which you were aware of the tension your partner was creating. Then think about what you experienced during that time, both physically and emotionally. Below are some examples of things that women describe about their experience during the tension phase of the Cycle. Look down the list and see if you have had any of these experiences.

During the Tension Phase, I...

- [ ] try to keep the peace
- [ ] keep busy
- [ ] keep the kids quiet
- [ ] cover up for the kids
- [ ] become forgetful
- [ ] have problems focusing
- [ ] worry
- [ ] feel fearful
- [ ] second guess myself
- [ ] wonder if I should leave
- [ ] think I've made a big mistake
- [ ] make lists to try to keep track of everything
- [ ] feel like a fool
- [ ] feel resigned to the situation
- [ ] feel hurt
- [ ] feel isolated
- [ ] feel exhausted
- [ ] feel irritated

- [ ] feel angry
- [ ] cry a lot
- [ ] have a knot in my stomach
- [ ] have pains in my chest
- [ ] have anxiety attacks
- [ ] feel depressed
- [ ] have nightmares
- [ ] have blurred vision
- [ ] over eat/under eat
- [ ] can't sleep/sleep too much
- [ ] retreat into myself
- [ ] think about death as a way to escape
- [ ] feel like I can't make a decision
- [ ] _____
- [ ] _____
- [ ] _____
- [ ] _____

As you can see from the list, living with constant tension has a devastating effect on your health and well-being as well as on your ability to make decisions that will help keep you safe.

Why is the explosion so awful?

Now let's think about what happens to you during the explosion phase of the Cycle. For many women, this is the most frightening time in the Cycle. Although men are not out of control, they may appear to be out of control and that is frightening. If your partner is driving recklessly, throwing something in your direction, startling you out of sleep, humiliating you with words or attacking you physically or sexually, your well-being as a person is being seriously threatened.

As well as being frightened during this phase, women also find the explosion affects their self-identity. The explosions can humiliate and degrade you. If you are told that you are stupid or selfish or a bitch, this will obviously undermine your sense of self-worth. It is difficult to feel positive or realistic about yourself when your self-identity is always being attacked.

One of the very destructive aspects of the explosion phase is that you are being blamed for the explosion. This can also affect your self-identity and your sense of reality. Let's use an example to illustrate this.

Emily

Emily, who is married and has two children, is invited by her fellow employees to join them for drinks after work one night. She decides she would like to go. After carefully considering when it would be best to raise this with her partner, she asks him the night before. Emily asks if he could be home from work in time to relieve the baby sitter so Emily can go out. She also asks him to make the kids dinner and to watch them until she gets home. He chooses to explode in response to her request. He tells her that she's being self-centred. He reminds her that he has been working hard lately and the last thing he needs is to come home to baby-sit the kids. Besides, doesn't she think her kids deserve a piece of her too? After all, they are stuck with a sitter all day. He also accuses her of being interested in one of her colleagues and suggests that she may be having an affair. Emily is being falsely accused by her partner. Because she is interested in making her marriage work, however, she tries to sort through each of his accusations to see if they hold any truth. She wonders "Am I being selfish? Have I not paid enough attention to the stress my partner is living with? Am I not giving my kids enough time? Am I being flirtatious at work?"

Being forced to do this evaluation of herself causes a woman to keep the focus of the problem on her rather than on her partner's abuse. The result is that women often try to figure out how to stop the abuse in the explosion phase by changing themselves.

But no matter how much of the blame you have accepted and how much you have sought solutions, your partner continues the Cycle of Abuse. The abuse is not your fault. Below is a list of things women have experienced during the explosion phase of the Cycle. See if anything seems familiar to you.

During the Explosion Phase, I...

- ☐ feel scared
- ☐ try to get away
- ☐ feel trapped
- ☐ feel hopeless
- ☐ feel degraded
- ☐ become very quiet
- ☐ avoid eye contact
- ☐ shake
- ☐ give in to him
- ☐ try to end the relationship
- ☐ try to protect myself
- ☐ fight back

- ☐ yell
- ☐ feel like I'm going crazy
- ☐ swear
- ☐ hit him
- ☐ hit myself
- ☐ throw things
- ☐ shut myself off
- ☐ experience physical injuries
- ☐ _____
- ☐ _____
- ☐ _____
- ☐ _____

The explosion phase is a time of high stress because of the fear you feel. This affects you both physically and psychologically. As a society, we tend to associate the explosion with physical injury and that is sometimes the case. However, women are inevitably harmed psychologically by the explosion phase and that harm is often invisible and long-lasting. These are only some of the ways you may be affected by your partner's explosions.

What is my experience of the Cycle?

In our group counseling with women, we sketch out the Cycle of Abuse first from the perspective of the man's behaviour (as we did in chapter 2). Then we sketch out the Cycle from the point of view of the woman's experience. Drawing on all of the experiences of the women in the room, we come up with a Cycle that looks something like the one below. When you look at this Cycle, do not be concerned if some of your experience is not represented here; this is only an example.

Diagram 3.1   Women's Experience of the Cycle of Abuse

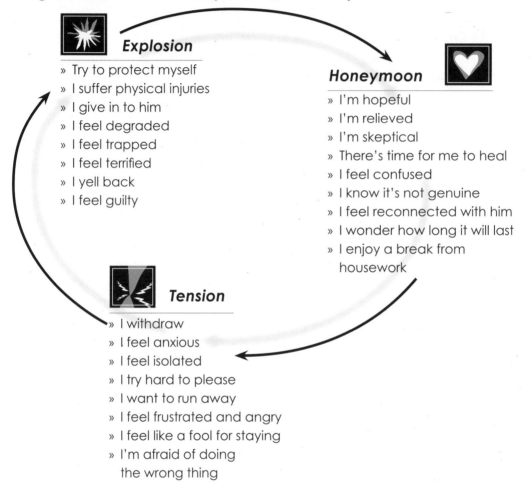

Explosion
- » Try to protect myself
- » I suffer physical injuries
- » I give in to him
- » I feel degraded
- » I feel trapped
- » I feel terrified
- » I yell back
- » I feel guilty

Honeymoon
- » I'm hopeful
- » I'm relieved
- » I'm skeptical
- » There's time for me to heal
- » I feel confused
- » I know it's not genuine
- » I feel reconnected with him
- » I wonder how long it will last
- » I enjoy a break from housework

Tension
- » I withdraw
- » I feel anxious
- » I feel isolated
- » I try hard to please
- » I want to run away
- » I feel frustrated and angry
- » I feel like a fool for staying
- » I'm afraid of doing the wrong thing

Looking at the Cycle as a whole, you can appreciate how confusing and complex the Cycle really is. Although everything that occurs in the Cycle is part of the abuse, women tend to experience a wide range of emotions and reactions as their partners are abusive in very different ways throughout the Cycle.

You might want to see what the Cycle looks like for you by taking the Cycle below and putting examples of things you have experienced. You can take some examples from the lists in this chapter and put them in the appropriate phases. This might help you to create a picture of what's going on for you as your partner continues to control you and your relationship through the Cycle of Abuse.

The Cycle of Abuse: Impact on Me

Explosion

Honeymoon

Tension

The Cycle affects each woman differently. Hopefully you are beginning to see for yourself how your partner's abusive behaviour during each phase of the Cycle affects you and how the Cycle overall impacts you in a very negative way.

You may have many reactions to what you have read in this chapter. Looking at the Cycle you've created may be overwhelming, liberating or both. Up until this point, you have not been able to pay much attention to yourself or the larger pattern of the relationship. You have been forced to put all your attention on your partner in hopes of diminishing or stopping the abuse. Focusing on his immediate needs, moods and demands may not give you the opportunity to see how his abuse is affecting you.

It may make you very sad, or angry, or frightened to realize that there is a pattern to the abuse you've experienced. It may also be very liberating, especially if you have felt that you are "going crazy" because your emotions or life seem out of control. Hopefully, you are beginning to see that you are not crazy, but your partner's behaviour is certainly crazy-making. We will look more closely at the effect your partner's abuse is having on you in chapter 5. Now let's turn our attention to the different kinds of abuse you may be experiencing.

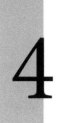

4

What are the different types of abuse?

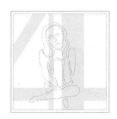

I remember him being angry. He pulled all of my clothes out of the closet and threw them on the floor. Then he pulled out all the drawers from my dresser. The whole time he kept yelling at me and telling me I was stupid. I was so overwhelmed and frightened I went into our spare room and just cried. He came in and tried to console me. I was so hurt, angry and humiliated—I just kept crying. In the morning I cleaned up the mess. I wondered what my little girl thought. I didn't say anything to him for fear of making him mad again. He acted like it had never happened, so I had to do the same. And life went on. **Jen**

How do I experience abuse?

Abuse takes many forms. No one type of abuse is worse than another type. All abuse has a negative impact on women.

What we hear from women who are abused is that emotional and verbal abuse is extremely difficult and painful, with long-term effects. Emotional abuse tends to be difficult to identify and name. It also tends to be pervasive in our society and thus may be more "acceptable" than other types of abuse. Despite women's experiences, many people think that physical abuse is the worst type and some believe it is the only type of abuse.

No one but you can assess how your partner's abuse has affected you or what types of abuse are most painful. We will further explore the effects of the abuse in chapter 5. For now, let's look at the many ways that women experience abuse from their intimate partners.

What is the Power and Control Wheel?

In order to examine the types of abuse, we will use something called the Power and Control Wheel.[1] The Wheel is divided into sections. Each section is given a heading of a category of abuse. Examples of that category are listed inside the wheel. We call these different examples of abuse the types or "tactics" of that category. At the centre of the wheel is written "Power and Control." This indicates that all tactics of abuse are used to maintain power and control in the relationship. No matter what tactics your partner uses, the effect is to control and intimidate you or to make you feel that you do not have an equal voice in the relationship.

Diagram 4.1 Power and Control Wheel

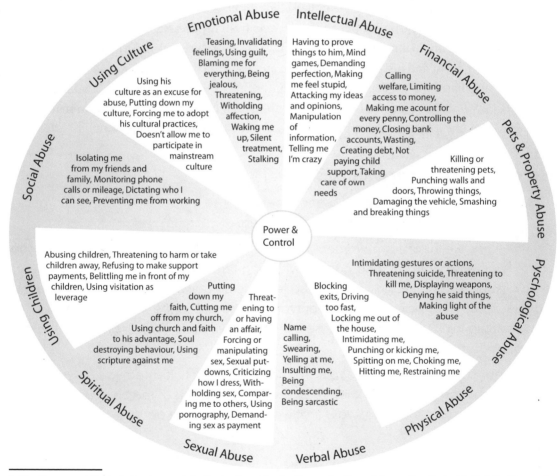

---

1 The Power and Control wheel was originally developed by the Domestic Abuse Intervention Project in Duluth, Minnesota. Our wheel is adapted from the original with permission.

What are the types of abuse?

It is difficult with one small Power and Control Wheel to list all the different types of abuse. A more complete list that summarizes many women's experiences is provided below. Each section begins with a brief description of the category of abuse.

We invite you to look down these lists and check off any kind of abuse you feel you have experienced. You may find that you check off more under one category than another. You may also find that you do not check off anything in some categories. You may want to add to this list from your own experience. Each woman's experience is unique.

Psychological/Mental Abuse

Any act intended to undermine your mental well-being.

☐ telling me I'm crazy

☐ giving me the silent treatment

☐ manipulating me

☐ playing mind games

☐ wearing down my instincts

☐ watching

☐ stalking

☐ distorting reality

☐ bringing up the past to deflect the issue at hand

☐ using information against me

☐ rewriting history

☐ intimidating or threatening me and claiming he's "just joking"

☐ putting on a good show to win others to his side

☐ giving me glaring looks

☐ making me prove things to him

☐ demanding perfection

☐ changing the rules

☐ _____

☐ _____

☐ _____

Physical/Threat of Physical Abuse

Any unwanted physical contact or threat of physical contact.

- [ ] making threatening gestures
- [ ] driving recklessly
- [ ] throwing things at me or near me
- [ ] restraining me
- [ ] blocking my exit from the room
- [ ] pushing, shoving, hitting, slapping, punching
- [ ] using weapons to threaten me or the children
- [ ] spitting
- [ ] choking
- [ ] pulling my hair

- [ ] biting or pinching
- [ ] kicking
- [ ] grabbing or shaking
- [ ] locking me out of the house
- [ ] threatening to kill me
- [ ] _____
      _____
- [ ] _____
      _____
- [ ] _____
      _____

Verbal Abuse

Any use of words or volume of voice to threaten, belittle or injure you.

- [ ] yelling or screaming
- [ ] name calling
- [ ] putting me down
- [ ] swearing
- [ ] using "sarcasm" & hurtful" jokes"
- [ ] saying "you always..." or "you never..."
- [ ] blaming me

- [ ] being condescending
- [ ] _____
      _____
- [ ] _____
      _____
- [ ] _____
      _____

Sexual Abuse

Any unwanted sexual contact.

☐ ridiculing me for saying "no"

☐ using my past sexual experience against me

☐ insisting on using pornography

☐ having or threatening to have an affair

☐ coercing sex by guilt, harassment or threats

☐ forcing sex (rape)

☐ criticizing how I dress (too sexy or not sexy enough)

☐ telling me I'm not "good enough"

☐ telling me I'm fat and undesirable

☐ putting me down sexually (e.g., calling me whore, slut, frigid, prude, etc.)

☐ demanding sex as payment

☐ talking to others about our sex life

☐ _____

☐ _____

☐ _____

☐ _____

Spiritual Abuse

Any word or action that damages you spiritually.

☐ using religious authority against me

☐ attacking my beliefs

☐ using scripture against me

☐ isolating me from my religious community

☐ destroying my soul

☐ _____

☐ _____

☐ _____

Using Children

Any involvement or use of children in the abuse.

☐ belittling me in front of children

☐ using children to his advantage

☐ threatening to take children from me

☐ fighting me for custody of the children

☐ not paying child support

☐ telling me I'm a terrible mother

☐ abusing the children

☐ threatening to harm the children

☐ using visitation to harass me

☐ _____

☐ _____

☐ _____

Social Abuse

Any attempt to cut you off from sources of support and care.

☐ isolating me

☐ cutting me off from friends

☐ embarrassing me in front of others

☐ controlling who I spend time with

☐ refusing to spend time with the family

☐ being jealous

☐ criticizing family members and friends so I stop seeing them

☐ monitoring phone calls

☐ monitoring car mileage

☐ preventing me from working

☐ _____

☐ _____

☐ _____

Cultural Abuse

Any use of cultural ideas as a way to dominate you.

☐ using culture to legitimize
abusive behaviour

☐ _____

☐ putting down my culture

☐ _____

☐ forcing me to adopt his cultural practices

_____

☐ speaking his language to exclude me

☐ _____

☐ using extended family to oppress me

_____

☐ refusing to allow me to learn
mainstream culture

_____

Emotional Abuse

Any act intended to undermine your emotional well-being.

☐ teasing

☐ invalidating my feelings

☐ trying to tell me how to feel

☐ blaming me for everything

☐ putting me in a "no win" situation

☐ withholding affection

☐ using a threatening tone of voice

☐ waking me up

☐ being jealous

☐ threatening suicide

☐ intimidating me

☐ making light of the abuse

☐ changing mood quickly (e.g.,
from calm to anger)

☐ withdrawing emotionally

☐ _____

☐ giving mixed messages
(e.g., love and hate)

☐ _____

☐ behaving unpredictably

_____

☐ making me feel guilty

☐ _____

☐ being competitive

_____

Intellectual Abuse

Any act intended to make you question your intellectual ability.

- [ ] making me look stupid
- [ ] claiming superior intelligence
- [ ] correcting my grammar
- [ ] confusing me
- [ ] belittling my intellectual ability
- [ ] not letting me finish my sentences

- [ ] showing off his higher education
- [ ] _____
- [ ] _____
- [ ] _____

Financial Abuse

Any intentional act that deprives you (or your children) of financial security or limits your access to financial decision making.

- [ ] making me account for every cent
- [ ] making me justify every purchase
- [ ] withholding financial information
- [ ] hiding money from me
- [ ] limiting my access to money
- [ ] closing out joint bank accounts without my consent
- [ ] spending money needed for the household on himself (or gambling it away)
- [ ] belittling my financial contributions to the household
- [ ] threatening to take all the money if I should separate

- [ ] spending money carelessly
- [ ] making me beg for money
- [ ] forcing me to commit welfare fraud
- [ ] threatening to call welfare
- [ ] leaving me with the burden of paying bills when there's not enough money
- [ ] making financial decisions without me
- [ ] not paying child support
- [ ] _____
- [ ] _____
- [ ] _____

- ☐ running up bills
- ☐ forcing me to ask for a raise at work

_____

_____

Abuse of Pets and Property

Hurting pets or damaging property in order to intimidate, control and hurt you.

☐ threatening to hurt pets	☐ breaking treasured items
☐ punching walls and doors	☐ _____
☐ killing pets	_____
☐ throwing things	☐ _____
☐ damaging the vehicle	_____
☐ smashing things	

What is his motive?

It's important here to say a word about motives. As you looked down these lists, you may have discovered behaviours that you have resorted to yourself. Please look at these behaviours within the context of your motives. Let's take an obvious example to illustrate our point.

We've said that physical abuse is any form of unwanted physical touch. However, without some consideration of motives, this definition suggests that stepping on someone's toe accidentally is a form of abuse. It is, after all, unwanted physical contact. Yet, if you step on someone's toe accidentally, your motive is not to control or to intimidate him or her. The physical contact is accidental; his or her toe just happened to be where you set your foot down.

Similarly, in an attempt to get away from your partner who is yelling at you and blocking your exit from a room, you may push him. This is unwanted physical contact from his point of view, but it is not your intention to control him or to have power over him. You are simply trying to remove yourself from a situation that is not safe for you, either physically or emotionally. Your motive is self-protection, not gaining power and control over your partner.

Often women will describe their motive as simply wanting to be heard and respected—they want to be treated as an equal by their partner. Sometimes women do yell at, swear at or hit their partners. When women explore the motives behind their behaviour, they discover that their ideas, opinions or feelings have not been acknowledged. Their actions are a response to being repeatedly silenced, a form of abuse that has a significant impact for women. One woman expressed her intentions this way:

> After several hours of grueling verbal attacks from my partner, I lost it. I walked in the house and he followed. I turned and began to hit him and scream. Then I realized that this was not me. I stopped, and started to cry. I did not do any of that to control him. I had not stooped to his level. I just wanted to be heard and still he was not hearing me. I realized then he would never hear my voice. For him, I had no voice. **Marie**

At the centre of the Power and Control Wheel is the phrase "Power and Control." All the abusive behaviours listed are intended to have the same effect—to control and intimidate. While Marie may have wanted some control in this particular situation, she was only interested in being heard. She did not want control over every aspect of the relationship. While her behaviour was not desirable, it was not abusive. Her motive was self-preservation.

Remember that such behaviour is potentially dangerous, as an abusive partner may have more physical, financial and social power than you do. Perhaps your partner has relentlessly attacked you and ridiculed you, to the point that you finally yell back, slam something down or even push him. You may feel a temporary sense of control or relief, but it could also further jeopardize your safety.

How can I make a Power and Control Wheel for myself?

On the following page is a Power and Control Wheel for you to complete. Your first step is to name the categories for yourself. Keep in mind that there is no "right" way to do this. For example, some women might combine emotional, intellectual and verbal abuse together into one category, while other women want to separate these out. Simply decide what categories work best for you.

There is also no "right" way to fill in the categories with examples of different tactics. If your partner has blocked your exit from the bathroom, you might describe this as physical abuse—it is physically threatening. You might also describe it as emotional abuse—he is holding you hostage. It is also sexual abuse—he is invading you in a physically private space. Simply list the tactic of abuse in whatever category works best for you. You may want to list a tactic or example in more than one category.

Power and Control Wheel

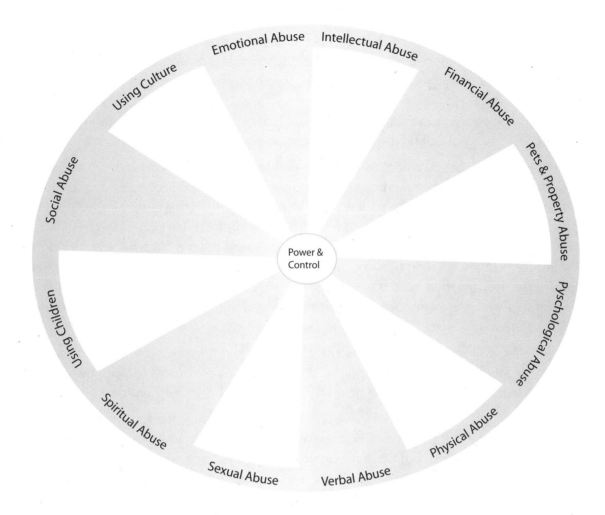

How might I feel after completing my Power and Control Wheel?

The Power and Control Wheel may have helped you to identify some of your experiences of abuse that you had not recognized before. For example, you might have recognized that your partner was physically and verbally abusive, but had more difficulty naming some of his behaviour as financially, intellectually or sexually abusive.

You may also feel quite overwhelmed at seeing how many kinds of abuse you checked off and how full your Wheel is. Women often say that they didn't realize how pervasive the abuse was until they had completed this exercise.

Women often find that the Power and Control Wheel clarifies why they were uncomfortable with some of their partner's seemingly acceptable behaviours. For example, if you manage the finances in your relationship, it appears that you have financial control. However, if your partner also monitors and criticizes you for the financial situation you are in, you aren't actually managing the budget. You are probably worrying about his reaction to your budgeting more than the budget itself.

The Power and Control Wheel may cause you to ask whether your partner's use of the tactics is intentional. You may also wonder how aware he is of trying to maintain his control in the relationship. At this point in our women's group, women frequently ask, "Does this mean he doesn't love me? Is he only interested in controlling me?" You are in the best position to answer this question, but one thing is clear: women tend to focus more on the relationship while men who are abusive focus more on their own needs. He may still love you, but maintaining his control is more important than the relationship. It can be very painful to recognize that your partner puts himself before you and the relationship.

While dealing with these difficult realizations, women often express relief because they can finally make sense of their partner's actions. Whatever you are feeling, be gentle with yourself; the process you are going through is shared by many women.

Before moving to the next chapter, we would like to summarize the four main purposes of the Power and Control Wheel. First, the Wheel helps you to identify forms or tactics of abuse that you might not have recognized as abuse. Second, the Wheel illustrates to you that the desire to maintain power and control in the relationship is central to your partner's motives. Third, you may have minimized or disregarded many of these behaviours because, taken alone, they didn't seem that serious. The Wheel allows you to see that it is the sum of all these behaviours that has had an impact on you, and not the severity of any one incident of abuse. Finally, the list that you compiled shows the tactics your partner uses to intimidate and control you. Hopefully, this list will help you to understand the intent behind your partner's behaviour.

In the next chapter we will look at the extent to which, and in what ways, the abuse is affecting you.

5

What's the abuse doing to me?

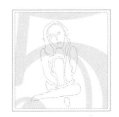

> Within six months of leaving my husband, Jeff, I was able to stop taking my blood pressure medication. I always thought that this was a permanent condition. I also believed that I had high blood pressure because I couldn't cope with stress. I never thought that it was because of the constant fear and tension of living with an unpredictable and abusive man. **Claire**

Although Claire was never physically assaulted by her partner, the emotional abuse was constant. Every day he found some reason to be critical and argumentative. The stress of living with Jeff took a huge toll on Claire's health.

How serious is the abuse?

The seriousness of the abuse cannot be judged by the type of abuse you are experiencing, but rather by the impact it is having on you. Often the impact of the abuse is a result of the ongoing, unpredictable, seemingly random actions and reactions of your partner. This reality is invisible to most people. You have probably done a good job of concealing the difficulties you face in your relationship, especially if you have been told the problem is yours. Many women in our groups begin by minimizing or downplaying the abuse. They will say, "It's not that bad. He's never actually hit me. It's mostly been verbal abuse." This type of statement underestimates the harm that all forms of abuse can have on you.

Our society tends to recognize physical abuse because it is perceived to be the most threatening to women. Physical violence is serious and can lead to very painful and even permanent injuries. However, we also want to take seriously the impact of other types of abuse. Let's look at four examples that illustrate the impact of other forms of abuse.

Sandra

Jim and Sandra have a disagreement while in the car. Jim drives recklessly, causing Sandra to feel fearful and back down from the argument. Jim does not intend to physically harm Sandra—he only wants to frighten her. However, his recklessness does, in fact, end in an accident. Sandra sustains injuries, including a broken wrist. Do you think the impact on Sandra is any different than if Jim had broken her wrist during an assault?

Brenda

Dave and Brenda have a disagreement while in the living room. Dave becomes more and more enraged and will not let Brenda leave the room. He finally throws a book at Brenda, which misses her head by only inches. Do you think the impact of this incident is different for Brenda than if Dave had actually hit her head?

Reena

Rajiv and Reena have been together since they were teenagers. Rajiv has never hit Reena, but he is unrelenting in his emotional attacks. He is critical of her appearance and of everything she does. Rajiv's abuse has caused Reena to develop anorexia nervosa. Reena may be starving herself to death. How would you assess the lethality of Rajiv's abuse?

Charlene

Ray has closed all the bank accounts and Charlene does not know what he has done with their money. He gives her a limited "allowance" to take care of all of the household needs. She is unable to meet all the financial demands that are placed on her as she tries to provide for their three children. Charlene has a serious heart condition that has always been monitored by her doctor, and with the new financial stresses placed on Charlene because of Ray's abuse, her heart condition has worsened. Her doctor urges her to remove all sources of stress from her life, but Ray refuses all the suggestions she offers to improve the situation. How lethal do you think this situation is?

These scenarios point to an important truth. Abusive men do not need to be physically violent to be abusive. None of the men in these scenarios hit their partner, but the impact of the abuse is quite profound.

No matter how much we counter the cultural idea that only physical abuse is serious, many women still feel that the emotional, verbal, financial and spiritual abuse isn't "that bad" and feel that they should be able to handle it. Taking the impact of all forms of abuse seriously will help to validate all you have been experiencing in your relationship.

What is the impact of the abuse?

In order to keep yourself (and your children) emotionally and physically safe, you've had to pay a great deal of attention to your partner. You probably carefully monitor your partner's moods and behaviour. You may not have had much opportunity to see how his abuse affects you.

When we work with women in group counseling, we invite them to list the ways that their partners' abuse has affected them. We ask them what impact the abuse has had on them. The women brainstorm and fill several pages of flip chart paper with examples of how they have been affected by the abuse.

Below is a list generated by a group of women of the impact the abuse had on them. The list covers every aspect of a woman's life—emotional, intellectual, physical, financial, social and spiritual. We invite you to read down the list and check off the ways in which you have been affected by your partner's abuse, and we encourage you to add to the list at the bottom.

Impact List

- [ ] wonder if I'm going crazy
- [ ] feel isolated
- [ ] suffer depression
- [ ] feel a lack of interest
- [ ] have no energy
- [ ] feel disillusioned
- [ ] feel distracted
- [ ] feel my work is affected
- [ ] feel overwhelmed
- [ ] want to avoid people/crowds
- [ ] lie to people: "I'm fine"

- [ ] have heart palpitations
- [ ] have high blood pressure
- [ ] have difficulty breathing
- [ ] have frequent headaches
- [ ] have recurring bladder infections
- [ ] have recurring yeast infections
- [ ] experience dizziness
- [ ] don't like myself
- [ ] feel ugly
- [ ] judge myself
- [ ] feel parts of my personality are flawed

- [ ] am forced to keep secrets
- [ ] feel a lack of support
- [ ] feel lonely
- [ ] feel suicidal
- [ ] am forgetful
- [ ] blank out/black out
- [ ] feel numb
- [ ] feel nervous
- [ ] fear being trapped
- [ ] experience an emotional roller coaster
- [ ] am afraid I won't get out safely
- [ ] feel vulnerable
- [ ] feel terrified
- [ ] have to justify myself/my time
- [ ] feel paranoid
- [ ] get panic attacks
- [ ] feel brainwashed
- [ ] feel anxious
- [ ] feel I have to look busy all the time
- [ ] feel on the alert all the time
- [ ] smoke more
- [ ] drink more alcohol
- [ ] drink more coffee
- [ ] use drugs more
- [ ] watch TV more
- [ ] gamble more

- [ ] don't value myself
- [ ] lose myself
- [ ] lose interest in physical/sexual intimacy
- [ ] stop doing what I enjoy
- [ ] don't think I deserve to have needs
- [ ] do everything for him (for safety)
- [ ] forget my needs
- [ ] am afraid to have my own life, friends
- [ ] have little self-respect
- [ ] feel guilt about him leaving/me leaving
- [ ] don't feel important
- [ ] feel like a failure
- [ ] feel incapable
- [ ] engage in self-monitoring and/or self-censoring
- [ ] am self-conscious
- [ ] question myself
- [ ] lose my instincts
- [ ] doubt myself
- [ ] have a hard time trusting men
- [ ] feel callous
- [ ] am angry at myself
- [ ] yell at children/pets
- [ ] feel angry
- [ ] want to hurt him
- [ ] feel rage

- [ ] experience insomnia
- [ ] sleep too much
- [ ] wake suddenly in the night
- [ ] wake up in sweats
- [ ] have bad dreams
- [ ] lose my appetite
- [ ] eat too much
- [ ] develop ulcers
- [ ] develop digestive problems
- [ ] experience muscular pain
- [ ] experience nausea
- [ ] experience vomiting
- [ ] experience diarrhea
- [ ] experience anorexia/bulimia
- [ ] feel exhausted all the time
- [ ] get ill often

- [ ] feel like a prostitute
- [ ] become bankrupt
- [ ] lose my home
- [ ] fall into poverty
- [ ] lose my church
- [ ] lose my faith
- [ ] have my creativity stifled
- [ ] adapt after a long time
- [ ] _____
- [ ] _____
- [ ] _____
- [ ] _____
- [ ] _____
- [ ] _____
- [ ] _____
- [ ] _____

Most women are shocked to see the many ways in which the abuse has affected them. This list can be very affirming, because it helps to explain concerns that you may have had over states such as forgetfulness, dizziness, sadness or confusion. It may also help you to understand why you're so exhausted—look at all that you've been coping with!

Am I being brainwashed?

Some women have told us they feel like they are being brainwashed by their partners. We believe this is an accurate description of what is going on. Indeed, many abusive men use brainwashing tactics to control their partners. These tactics, however, may be difficult to identify because they are less obvious. Parallels have been drawn by researchers between the tactics interrogators use in prisoner-of-war camps to brainwash their prisoners and the tactics some abusive men use to control their partners. For example, a common brainwashing technique is sleep deprivation, which is used in order to weaken a prisoner's mental and physical ability to resist. Here is an example of how sleep deprivation can be used as a means of maintaining control in an intimate relationship.

Colleen

Colleen is exhausted. For the third night in a row, her partner has kept her up until 2:00 a.m., berating her for making plans to spend a weekend with her family. This is a common occurrence for Colleen. Sometimes, just as she's falling off to sleep, he'll insist on discussing something with her. Colleen can't remember the last time she had enough sleep. She finds herself giving in more to her partner's demands as she is too exhausted to disagree.

Another common brainwashing technique is degradation and humiliation. Prisoners are belittled and shamed by their interrogators until they no longer stand up for themselves; to do so is too costly to their self-esteem. The fear of humiliation is a powerful tool in controlling someone. Here is an example of how one woman's partner used this technique.

Bethany

Russell is an opinionated person who is quite vocal about his ideas in social settings. Bethany is often embarrassed by the extreme statements that Russell makes at parties. On a number of occasions, Bethany has attempted to moderate Russell's extreme views with her own more moderate statements. Each time Bethany does this, however, Russell embarrasses her by implying she is stupid or lacking in education. Bethany decides to remain silent at parties.

A third brainwashing technique used to control prisoners is that of enforcing trivial demands. Interrogators insist that prisoners obey their every whim. Eventually the prisoners stop thinking for themselves and do whatever they are told. Here is an example of how this tactic can be used in a relationship where there is abuse.

Julia

Brent insists on keeping "everything in its place." Their house is spotless and every knickknack and appliance has a place where it belongs. Over time, Brent changes the rules about where things are to go and Julia spends a lot of energy trying to anticipate how he would like the home to look. Lately Julia feels panicked when she comes home from work and she second guesses every decision she makes.

The parallels between the tactics used by interrogators and the tactics used by abusive men point to the profound effect that mental and emotional abuse can have on an individual. You may wonder why we draw these parallels. You certainly aren't a prisoner of war. You may get up and go to work each day, conducting yourself competently and independently. You may have many friends with whom you stay in touch. You may be responsible for all the financial management in your family. We know how strong and capable women are who live with abuse. Not for a moment would we suggest that you are weak or incapable. In the same way, your partner's motives are probably not identical to those of an interrogator.

These examples illustrate, however, the serious nature of your experiences of mental and emotional abuse and identify common reactions to this abuse. They describe the impact that tactics such as induced exhaustion, threats of degradation or the enforcement of trivial demands may be having on your mental or physical well-being.

We also include this information to show you how, in a situation of danger, people are forced to behave in ways that conflict with their true self. Your self is not lost, but you bury it in order to protect yourself from the emotional, sexual, physical, mental and verbal attacks. You may also have to go along with your partner's needs and demands, even if your heart isn't in it. Some women have felt forced to break the law or compromise their values. Prisoners of war respond the same way: they modify their behaviour to keep themselves safe. As with prisoners of war, you have found strategies to keep your children and yourself as safe as possible in an unpredictable situation. Such strategies show wisdom and courage on your part.

Will I always feel this bad?

Once again, it may be overwhelming or liberating or both to look at the work you have done in this chapter. You may be overwhelmed at your discovery of how much your partner's abuse has affected you. You may feel very sad or angry. You may, however, feel liberated at discovering an explanation for some of the things you have been experiencing. It may be helpful to realize that the reasons you eat, sleep or drink too much can be found in the abuse you have been living with.

Your partner's abuse has had a serious impact on you, leaving you feeling tired, confused and perhaps even ill. Women wonder if they will always feel as bad as they do now. Most women find that, once they have a break from the abuse, many of the negative effects go away. Although it can sometimes take a few months, women have described being able to sleep properly once again or having their blood pressure go back down to normal.

We realize that it may not be possible right now to escape your partner's abuse either temporarily or permanently. However, there are some things you can do to try to take care of yourself and lessen the impact of the abuse. Some women do this by attending a women's support group in order to share their experiences. Other women take advantage of opportunities to have time for themselves, even if it means just taking the dog for a walk. One woman volunteers outside her home because she feels valued by the staff and other volunteers. Receiving affirmation from outside sources has helped to keep her partner's unrelenting criticism in perspective.

Take some time to appreciate your ability to survive such a difficult relationship, especially one that impacts you in so many ways. Realizing what a difficult situation you are in and taking care of yourself will not change the situation. However, focusing on yourself when you can may at least give you the energy to take on the larger challenges that face you.

If it seems impossible to find any time, or you feel too exhausted to do anything, please be patient with yourself. Not judging yourself is a very important way of taking care of yourself.

We will explore these ideas further in the next chapter as we look more deeply at what is happening to you in your relationship.

6

Am I responsible for the abuse?

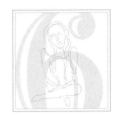

> I didn't like the way I behaved in my marriage. I always felt like I was "nagging" and making matters worse. I really tried hard to drop things or leave issues alone. I kept trying to change the way I was, believing that I was partly responsible for the mess we were in. **Janet**

Am I to blame?

Women often wonder if they are responsible for the problems in the relationship. They wonder if they are not coping well or if they are somehow making the situation worse. In this chapter, we hope to offer more positive ways of understanding yourself and how you are responding in your relationship. Let's look at some examples.

Pam

Pam has just finished reading another self-help book about relationships. She has been reflecting on the number of men that she has been with who have been hurtful to her, including her current partner. She is wondering if she's attracted to abusive men. With the help of the book she's reading, she has concluded that the abuse she experienced as a child has left her believing that abuse is normal in relationships. She decides that she must focus on healing herself from her past experiences.

Many self-help books are written primarily for women seeking answers to their own unhappiness, relationship problems or specific issues such as anger or intimacy. Many of these books assume that women are responsible for the problem. These books suggest that once a woman "fixes" herself, her relationship will be enhanced and the problems will disappear.

In concluding that she is attracted to abusive men, Pam is ignoring her partner's tactics in the honeymoon phase of the Cycle of Abuse. Her partner probably initially behaved in a respectful, considerate and intelligent manner, at which point Pam committed herself to the relationship. Pam saw qualities in her partner that were positive. These positive qualities attracted her to her partner, not the abuse.

If Pam thought abuse was normal, she would not be trying to bring about change in her relationship. She does know what qualities in a partner she wants and deserves, and she does not believe abuse is normal. Furthermore, if Pam does focus on her childhood experiences, she may be less guarded about her current safety. Such a focus allows her partner to exploit the idea that the problem lies in her "dysfunctional" childhood rather than in his need to control her. She is made to feel responsible for the difficulties in the relationship.

> As I began to look at sexual abuse from my past, my partner's abuse grew worse. I felt I was opening up a Pandora's box. He began to blame all the problems of our marriage on my dysfunctional childhood. The focus and blame switched to me. It kept him in control and me confused. After the divorce is final, I hope to be able to go back and heal from the sexual abuse and put those experiences behind me.   *Carla*

This book focuses not on your childhood experiences but rather on your current context of abuse. This is not because we wish to minimize the abuse you may have suffered in childhood or because we deem it unimportant, but because we believe it is more helpful to focus first and foremost on your current situation. It can be dangerous to focus too much on your childhood if you are with a partner who is abusive. You may reveal very painful stories to him only to have him use these against you. Being told that you deserved to be treated the way your mother treated you or having him re-enact something abusive your father did can be devastating. In the final analysis, whether or not you were abused as a child does not alter your current reality of abuse. You do not want your past to serve as an excuse for your partner's current behaviour. The focus needs to be on your partner and his responsibility for his behaviour. It can be dangerous if he places the responsibility on you.

Nancy

Nancy has been with her abusive partner for four years. She recently confided in a friend that she was very unhappy in her relationship. Her friend suggested that she is too focused on how she would like her partner to be and does not accept him as he is. Because of this, she is never satisfied. Nancy vows to be less critical of her partner. She also tells her mother about her resolve to be more supportive. Her mother enthusiastically supports her decision, stating that her partner works hard for his family and needs her unconditional support.

Nancy's friend fails to pay attention to the context in which Nancy lives, which is a context of abuse. Once we understand Nancy's experience in terms of the impact of abuse—her lack of freedom to express herself and her needs without being criticized and ridiculed—Nancy's need to focus on how she would like her partner to behave makes sense. While her friend has interpreted Nancy's behaviour as problematic, we understand Nancy's situation differently.

Nancy has clear and reasonable expectations of her partner—that he be respectful and contribute to the relationship. Indeed, she is focused on how she would like her partner to be because, as long as he is abusive, she is being hurt and oppressed. It makes sense to focus on his changing, because his current behaviour is unacceptable.

However, Nancy's partner perpetuates the idea that, if she were satisfied with the way things are, he wouldn't "lose his temper." Nancy then resolves to be less critical, hoping that this will solve the abuse and that he will not explode again. Nancy ends up taking responsibility for his behaviour.

Her mother's affirmation of Nancy's resolution to be more accepting of her partner conforms to many cultural assumptions about a woman's role in a relationship. Women are supposed to nurture their partner's ego and be unconditionally supportive. Furthermore, women are supposed to be grateful for a man's attention, however limited that is. If women "complain," they are unfeminine, selfish, demanding and hard to please. The cultural assumption is that men are abusive because their partners are uncooperative or too demanding. This assumption leaves women feeling responsible for the abuse.

Family and friends may blame women for the abuse in their relationship. They reinforce the idea that, if relationships are to improve, women must accommodate and compromise. This incorrect assumption presumes that women can effect change with a man whose primary interest is staying in control of the relationship. Trying harder may have some immediate benefits during the honeymoon phase, but these changes tend to be temporary. Nothing a woman does will make a lasting difference unless her partner is willing to let go of his desire for power and control.

Sandra

Sandra is feeling unappreciated in her relationship. She finds her partner is often disrespectful of her. She finally persuades him to go with her for marriage counseling. The therapist focuses on Sandra's behaviour and suggests that she does not have very good boundaries for herself. Sandra is told that she needs to get a lot clearer with her partner about what is disturbing for her in the relationship. He suggests she needs to be a lot more assertive and say "no" to her partner's criticisms and unreasonable demands. The therapist believes that Sandra's low self-esteem is the source of the problem. Sandra and her partner leave the counselor's office and return two weeks later. Sandra now describes an instance in which she tried to be more assertive. Her partner didn't speak to her for two days. The therapist states that perhaps Sandra was too aggressive in making her needs known. Furthermore, change is difficult, asserts the therapist, and so her partner was just reacting normally to a change in their communication patterns.

Many of the observations we made about Nancy's situation also apply to Sandra. Let's focus specifically on the advice Sandra received about setting boundaries. We think that Sandra has been very wise because she knows that saying "no" or trying to set boundaries is unsafe. With a partner who is respectful, of course, women can expect to set boundaries without consequence (although there is usually less need to do so in a respectful relationship). However, when a partner intends to remain in charge, he perceives her saying "no" as a threat to his control. He is likely to attack the "boundary" in order to regain control.

Sandra needed her counselor to affirm that it wasn't safe to set boundaries and that boundaries are not the issue. She had shown great wisdom and insight in the past by not asserting herself and her needs. While she has every right to express herself, as long as her partner is abusive, she will have to conceal herself and her needs. Sandra has experienced the consequences of disagreeing with him, expressing her opinion or saying "no" to something he is doing. She may never have felt physically threatened by her partner, but the emotional attacks on her self-identity make her fear his unpredictable responses. This lack of safety to express herself forces Sandra to use strategies to keep herself protected, sometimes even prompting Sandra to say and do things that are against her own values and principles. Again, some would interpret this as "unassertive" or "cowardly" behaviour on Sandra's part because she does not stand up for what she believes in, but we know Sandra has made a wise choice within the context of abuse. We understand Sandra's timid behaviour not as the cause of the abuse but rather as part of the impact of living with an abusive man.

As you can see by these examples, the problem is often interpreted as a weakness or deficit in the woman when the impact of abuse is not taken into account, such as Pam's childhood abuse, or Nancy's criticism of her partner. Often what women like Sandra have consciously or unconsciously used as a safety strategy, such as not setting limits or saying "no" to her partner, is misinterpreted as her problem.

One final assumption we challenge is the notion that Sandra's low self-esteem causes the abuse. Many women have been convinced that low self-esteem is the problem. We believe that the reverse is true—your partner's abuse has had an impact on you, and that affects how you feel about yourself. The problem is the abuse. You might ask yourself, "Did I feel better about myself before I was involved with this partner or at the beginning of this relationship?" Of course, if you have been with other abusive men, your self-esteem has probably already taken a battering.

Is there another way to look at my behaviour?

We would like to introduce another exercise intended to help you to "reframe" some of the ways in which you (or others) have interpreted your motives and behaviour. By reframing we mean offering you a different way to think about your behaviour. For example, if you have been told you are "not assertive enough," reframing helps you to understand this differently and say, "I need to be cautious in my relationship."

The Reframing Exercise describes "your problem" in a new light. It offers three alternative explanations for women's reaction to abuse: safety strategy, strength and impact.

This exercise will help you to see that much of your behaviour is a safety strategy, designed to keep you safe. You may also realize that what you do shows great strength of character on your part rather than demonstrating some sort of problem or shortcoming. Finally, some of what you do may simply be a result of the abuse or the impact of the abuse.

In the chart below we first list negative ideas that women sometimes have about themselves or that are suggested to them by others. We then offer alternative ways of understanding these feelings and behaviours. We have left blank spaces at the end of the chart for you to write additional descriptions of your motives and behaviour, either held by you or placed on you by others. These descriptions imply that you are responsible for the problem. Reframing them to reflect a more accurate interpretation of your intentions will help you to see that your behaviour is not the problem that your partner would have you believe. Instead, you will see that you have been acting wisely in a situation of abuse.

Diagram 6.1   Reframing Exercise

Negative Description	Safety Strategy	Strength	Impact
"You're a trouble maker"	I need to defend myself against my partner's accusations	I have my own opinions and ideas	I'm made to feel responsible for problems
"You can't handle conflict"	I watch out for my emotional and physical well-being	I'm able to negotiate and compromise in my relationships	My experiences of abuse have made me afraid of conflict
"You're too dependent on your partner"	I know my independence threatens my partner's need to control me	I'm interested in my partner and our relationship	My partner has forced me to be dependent (socially, financially, etc.)
"Your expectations are too low"	I know it is unsafe to state my expectations	I am a tolerant person	My partner does not meet my expectations so I am forced to lower them
"You are not assertive enough"	I know it is unsafe to express my needs or opinions	I am respectful of others	My experiences of abuse have made me cautious
"You nag too much"	I know I have to remind my partner or I will be blamed for his forgetfulness	I'm asking my partner to be responsible for his part in the relationship	I have to repeat myself in order to be heard
"You love too much"	I have to be loving so he won't become angry and abusive	I am a caring, compassionate person	The honeymoon phase of the Cycle keeps me engaged in the relationship
"You pay too much attention to your partner's feelings"	I focus on my partner's moods to anticipate explosions	I care about my partner	I am unable to pay attention to my personal needs

Negative Description	Safety Strategy	Strength	Impact

Hopefully, the Reframing Exercise has helped you to appreciate your strengths, despite the fact that some people may see them as faults. Sometimes other people, even if they care for you, do not understand the context of abuse and the importance of using strategies and wisdom to protect yourself and your children.

The following example further illustrates how some "solutions" can be dangerous. Here is what one woman was instructed to do by her therapist (who knew she lived with an abusive partner):

> **Therapist**: When he gets angry, you've got to just step up to the line and assert yourself. Don't let him push you off that line.

The therapist holds the following assumptions:

▶ The woman is responsible for the problem.

▶ She's not assertive enough.

▶ She lets herself be pushed around.

▶ Her partner gets upset and she backs away. He's learned he can get away with this behaviour. It is her responsibility to teach him he can't.

▶ She's letting her partner take advantage of her and take control. If she takes control, he'll respect her more (i.e., he won't be angry).

Perhaps you have heard the messages of responsibility so often that they feel like your own ideas. This woman accepted the following ideas as her own, even though they put her at risk:

▶ I need to try harder.

▶ I should understand what he's going through.

▶ He's in pain too—I need to be more patient.

▶ I've got to make this work.

▶ If only I were stronger.

▶ If only I had higher self-esteem.

▶ If only I were more assertive.

▶ I need to focus on the future rather than holding on to the past.

In contrast to the therapist, here's how we might interpret this woman's intentions and behaviours if we assume she is wise and acting strategically:

▶ She has already tried in hundreds of ways to prevent or decrease his anger and the response is always abusive.

▶ She is smart to move away from "the line" in a confrontation because she has been injured physically and emotionally when she has tried to defend herself.

▶ She has the right to assert herself, but for her safety she chooses to go along with her partner's demands.

The therapist in this case was irresponsible. He did not believe that the woman was at risk, and because she was willing to try any suggested action to stop the abuse, she was easy to work with. We hope that this story will give you the affirmation and courage you need to disregard the advice of anyone who doesn't believe your experience and affirm you in your decisions.

We encourage you to continue using the Reframing Exercise to understand your experiences. Practice making a mental "flip" whenever someone offers an explanation or description of you that suggests you are the problem. Ask yourself, "Is there a more accurate way to describe my motives and behaviour that includes the impact of the abuse?"

So who is responsible?

This chapter may have been difficult for you to work through. If you have always believed that you were responsible for the problems in the relationship, it can be challenging to start thinking in a new way. As a woman, you were raised to pay a lot of attention to others and to your relationship. You know how to take care of the people around you. Because of this you have always been very willing to work on your relationship and to take responsibility for your actions. The end result is that you may have accepted more than your share of the blame.

Until now you may have felt that, since the problem lies with you, you have some power to change it. But no matter what you have done to deal with a problem, your partner has sabotaged it, undermined your efforts, distorted the reality or shifted the problem back on to you. It is painful to realize that you do not have the power to stop your partner's abuse. Only he has the ability to stop being abusive.

We are not suggesting that women do not hold any responsibility for the problems in their relationship. What we are suggesting is that, as long as you are living with abuse, everything you do must be about staying safe and trying to keep peace in your relationship. Only when you are completely safe in your relationship can you explore relationship issues such as conflict resolution, open communication, your sexual relationship or issues from your childhood.

We have spent the first six chapters talking about your partner's behaviour and your experiences of abuse. While you may be gaining a clearer picture of the different kinds of abuse your partner employs and the affect this abuse has on you, you no doubt have deeper questions you would like to address. Most women want to know why their partner behaves the way he does. Many women also ask questions about how the abuse is affecting their children. We will turn to these questions in the next two chapters.

7

Why is my partner abusive?

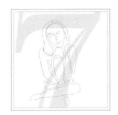

My husband insisted that he could do the housework better than I could. When he did do the housework, he took all day and ignored everything and everyone else. He wouldn't respond to the kids, and we were just supposed to stay out of his way. Then he insisted that we keep the house clean, with nothing out of place. With two young children, this was an impossible expectation. The clean house was just another way to show me he was superior and was also an excuse to verbally attack me when it got messy. *Patricia*

Why is my partner like this?

No doubt you have spent a lot of time and energy trying to figure out what causes your partner to behave the way he does. Listed below are some common explanations women struggle with as they try to make sense of their partner's behaviour. Some may sound familiar to you.

1. My partner has a problem with his anger (or has a bad temper) and sometimes he simply loses control.

2. My partner lives with a lot of stress because of his work (or lack of work) and his explosions are a result of this stress.

3. My partner suffers from some form of mental illness (depression, schizophrenia, personality disorder). He can't help the way he behaves.

4. My partner was abused as a child and is repeating patterns.

5. My partner is addicted to drugs or alcohol and would stop being abusive if he were clean and sober.

6. My partner and I have different styles for dealing with conflict.

Although these are common explanations in our culture, they probably do not account for your partner's behaviour. Indeed, your partner may be stressed or depressed or come from an abusive or dysfunctional home, but none of these explanations fully describes or justifies your partner's abusive behaviour. Let's look more closely at each of them.

1. My partner has a problem with anger.

It is a common idea that abusive men have a problem with anger and therefore simply lose control sometimes and become abusive. You can test this theory by thinking about a time when your partner was angry at someone else and yet didn't become abusive. For example, has your partner ever been angry with his boss and become abusive? Would he treat his boss with the same level of abuse he directs towards you?

Most women know that their partners would never swear at, yell at or hit a boss or co-worker. If your partner is able to "control" himself in his work place, he is able to control himself at home. Although your partner's behaviour may seem to be out of control, he is actually using his anger to intimidate you and regain control over you.

2. My partner lives with a lot of stress.

Your partner may live with a lot of stress. These days, many people do. Stop and think about all the sources of stress in your life (e.g., work, parenting, household responsibilities, extended family, dealing with an abusive man). Even though you also live with stress, you are not being abusive. Living with stress is never an excuse for being abusive.

3. My partner is mentally ill.

Sometimes women think their partner must be mentally ill because his behaviour is so bizarre or erratic. Some abusive men are even diagnosed by doctors or counselors with some form of mental illness. Ask yourself two questions: First, does your partner display this "abnormal" behaviour with everyone or just with you? Is he depressed around or paranoid with other people? If he does not consistently display "abnormal" behaviour, he may not be mentally ill.

Second, does having a mental illness give someone permission to be abusive? In our work with women, we find that many of them struggle with depression and yet they are not abusive. Having a mental illness and being abusive are two separate issues.

4. My partner was abused as a child.

It is tragic if your partner was abused as a child. But that is no excuse for his abusing you. What he does now is his choice. He is responsible for his behaviour. Do you know of others who were abused as children yet who are not abusive to their partners (e.g., a friend or yourself)? Sadly, many people were abused as children. However, we are not doomed to repeat the failures of our parents.

5. My partner is addicted to drugs or alcohol.

If your partner has an addiction, that is a serious problem. His abuse, however, is a separate issue. Many women have found that even after their partner "sobers up," he continues to be abusive.

6. My partner has a different style for dealing with conflict than I do.

Abuse is never an acceptable "style" of conflict resolution. Conflict means disagreement. Both partners have an equal opportunity to express themselves, without fear of the repercussions. When two people try to resolve conflict, neither leaves the discussion feeling attacked, intimidated or humiliated. It's not conflict if you feel attacked and silenced—it's abuse.

We've spent a lot of time explaining what abusive behaviour is not. Here is an alternative explanation with which many women and their partners agree.

What belief system is held by abusive men?

A study conducted at the University of British Columbia offers an insightful explanation for abusive men's behaviour. Through their extensive interviews with abusive men, researchers found that these men consistently communicated similar beliefs and ideas. The beliefs they held supported their actions to maintain power and control over their partner. [1]

The research pointed to three key ideas that make up the belief system of abusive men. Women have consistently expressed to us that these three ideas accurately reflect their partner's beliefs and behaviours. During the research process, many of the men were consulted after they completed a counseling group for men. The men confirmed that these were beliefs they held. The beliefs are:

---

1   M.N. Russell and J. Frohberg, Comparison of Confronting Abusive Beliefs and Anger Management Treatments for Assaultive Males (Vancouver: University of British Columbia, 1995).

- He is **Central** in the relationship.
- He is **Superior** in the relationship.
- He is **Deserving** of many privileges within the relationship.

In chapter 4, we stated that the purpose of your partner's behaviour is to maintain power and control over you. Now we want to explore the beliefs your partner holds that lead him to think he has a "right" to hold power and control over you. Let's look at each of these beliefs, along with some specific attitudes or behaviours that are a result of these beliefs. Not all of these examples will reflect your experience, but some may be familiar.

Central

- His work, hobbies and interests are more important than yours.
- His needs come before yours or your children's.
- He demands your attention whenever he wants it.
- He is active with the children, but only when he's interested.
- He does housework, and then expects a lot of praise.
- The household operates according to his timetable (e.g., dinner is ready when he wants it).
- Everything needs to be scheduled around his needs.

Superior

- In anything that is "important," he is better than you are.
- He criticizes you often.
- He thinks he is smarter than you are.
- His opinions are more valuable than yours.
- He thinks he is superior to other men.
- It is important that he makes more money than you.
- He devalues or dismisses what you do (at home or work).

Deserving

- He feels he has a right to rest or relaxation.
- He expects you to do more of the housework.
- He expects praise for every household task he does.
- He expects you to do more of the parenting.

> He expects sex whenever he wants it.

> He expects to be fed and cared for.

Abusive men will use any tactic to enforce their desire to be central, superior and deserving in the relationship. Let's look at some examples of how this belief system allows for his abusive behaviour.

Centrality

> **Darlene** and her two-year-old daughter, Christie, are sick with the flu. Because Darlene needs to go to bed, she asks Tom to stay up to care for their daughter. Tom has an early morning meeting and does not want to stay up late. Darlene tries to explain that she is really quite ill and unable to care for Christie.
>
> Tom becomes angry and accuses her of not being supportive of his work. Clearly she has no idea how demanding and stressful his job is. Why should he have to put up with more demands at home? She never thinks about anybody but herself. He suggests that she isn't really that sick and is just being selfish. When Darlene defends herself, Tom's abuse escalates until he calls her a "selfish bitch" and a "lazy mother." He storms out of the house and, when he returns, goes straight to bed. Darlene is left to care for Christie.

Because Tom thinks his needs are central, he puts himself before his partner's or his daughter's needs. Tom uses verbal accusations, threatening behaviour and name calling to avoid being responsible to his partner or his child and to maintain his centrality in the household.

Superiority

> **Gail** and Doug need a new vehicle. Gail looks in the paper every day for reasonably priced family cars and often points out cars that she thinks they can afford. Doug is never very interested in her suggestions. One day Doug comes home with a new truck. The truck cost significantly more than they had budgeted and it is not the "family car" Gail thought they had agreed to purchase.
>
> When Gail questions Doug's actions, he becomes defensive. She asks why they didn't go to look at some of the cars from the paper together. He tells her that she doesn't know anything about cars and everything she was looking at in the paper was "crap." When Gail discovers that the new truck means $300 a month in loan repayments, she becomes furious. She feels they are already burdened by too much debt. He tells her that, if she

wasn't such a wimp, she would ask her boss for a raise and then they wouldn't have any money problems.

Gail reminds Doug that their bad financial situation is a result of the debt he brought into the marriage. He is furious at her for "bringing up the past" and shoves her against the wall. She pushes him back and he grabs her hair and bangs her head into the wall. Frightened and hurt, Gail decides to drop it and leaves the room.

Doug's belief that he has a superior knowledge of vehicles allows him to make a unilateral decision and buy a truck without first consulting Gail. He also makes himself superior by belittling Gail's efforts and knowledge. Furthermore, by accusing Gail of being responsible for their financial difficulties, he shifts the problem to Gail's "inferior" ability to manage her work place. By accusing her of bringing up the past and physically abusing her, he silences Gail's protest. He can interpret this as "winning," thus ensuring his superior status. Doug uses financial, verbal and physical abuse to maintain his superiority.

Deserving

Tanya asks Greg if he has had any thoughts about his upcoming vacation time. She is hoping that the whole family can go camping together. Greg complains that such a trip would not be relaxing for him. He wants to take his two weeks and go fishing with some friends. Tanya reacts strongly to this idea. She wants some "family time" and doesn't want to be left alone with three children. He argues that he works hard and needs his vacation to be a vacation. She insists that she also works hard raising the children. He laughs at her and tells her that she doesn't know what hard work is.

Tanya suggests that he go fishing for part of the time but camp with the family for the remainder of his vacation. He tells her that if he can't go fishing for all of it, there's no point in going for any of it. Clearly feeling sorry for himself, Greg sulks for the next week and hardly speaks to Tanya or the children. As his vacation time approaches, Tanya realizes that he's going to make camping miserable for the family and suggests that he go on the fishing trip. He readily agrees and his mood immediately improves.

Greg believes that he deserves a vacation from all of life's responsibilities—something Tanya never gets to have. She is forced to put her needs aside because he considers them unimportant. Tanya and the children are not included in Greg's decision making because, from his perspective, only he deserves a holiday. He belittles Tanya's hard work and the needs of the family as a way of ensuring that he can justify his deservedness. Greg uses emotional abuse to get his way.

Why doesn't he treat me with respect?

It is normal for couples to disagree with each other from time to time, but the above examples demonstrate two main problems. First, the power and control belief system is about men being self-centred; this is not conducive to building respectful relationships.

Second, the man uses abusive tactics in order to impose his belief system. The abusive tactics allow him to stay in control and to have more power than his partner. An abusive man will use whatever forms of abuse he needs to "win" and get what he wants.

In contrast to the power and control belief system, which allows men to be central, superior and deserving, respectful individuals are interested in a "relationship" belief system. People living within a relationship belief system are interested in having

- ▶ *connection* with their partner;
- ▶ *equality* with their partner;
- ▶ *mutuality* with their partner.

The diagram below compares these two belief systems.

Diagram 7.1   Contrasting Belief Systems

Power and Control Belief System	← or →	Relationship Belief System
Central	← or →	Connected
Superior	← or →	Equal
Deserving	← or →	Mutual

Here are some attitudes or actions that reflect a relationship belief system:

Connected

- ▶ You make major decisions together.
- ▶ You enjoy activities together.

► The needs of the individual do not come at the expense of the family or the relationship.

Equal

► Each partner's needs are equally considered.

► The strengths of each partner are valued.

► Each partner is seen as intelligent and competent.

► The contributions of each partner are valued.

Mutual

► You share parenting and household responsibilities.

► You care for each other.

► You support each other's interests.

► You are respectful of each other.

Women, who are usually raised to consider the needs of others, often function out of this relationship belief. You have probably been approaching your relationship with the intention of being connected, equal and mutual.

It may be devastating for you to realize that you and your partner are working from two very different belief systems. You are working on creating a respectful and equal relationship. His primary concern has been with maintaining power and control and holding on to his superiority and privilege. You have been playing the game using different sets of rules and perhaps never knew it!

You have probably assumed that you and your partner share an interest in your relationship. Not only is this not true, but your partner assumes that you share his belief system. He believes you are also trying to be central, superior and deserving. Therefore, when you behave as his equal, he thinks you are trying to be better than he is. When you include your needs, he thinks you are being selfish. Abusive men often think that women are "out to get them" and that there is a "natural warfare" between the sexes. When men try to fight a war and women try to develop a relationship, women almost inevitably get hurt.

Furthermore, your partner's belief system forces you into a lesser role. If your partner insists on being central, you are forced into being peripheral. If your partner believes he is superior, then you must be inferior. If you partner is deserving, then you end up serving his needs. His belief system forces you into this behaviour. In order to protect yourself from further abuse, you are forced to accommodate his desire to be central, superior and deserving.

Diagram 7.2   Accomodating His Desire for Centrality

Your Partner	You
Central	Peripheral
Superior	Inferior
Deserving	Serving

Sometimes women try to share this information with their partner, in the hope that he will change his behaviour. However, your partner will likely disagree with the analysis. He will insist that he does not see himself as central, superior and deserving, in part because these beliefs are usually held unconsciously by abusive men. The beliefs are deep-seated, and your partner may not be entirely aware of them. As well, it is unlikely that he would admit to such selfish attitudes. Abusive men will rarely say that they are the "centre of the household" or "better than their partner" or "deserving of privileges." Their actions, however, betray their attitudes. If you want to test the theories of this chapter, we suggest you use your partner's behaviour as evidence, rather than what he says he believes.

> My partner always presented himself as being interested in "women's equality" and he "believed" he should do his share of housework. However, his behaviour betrayed a different set of beliefs. His constant criticisms pointed to his belief that he was superior to me. His disregard for my needs demonstrated his desire to be central and deserving. His actions were a better indication of his true belief system.   *Gabrielle*

Is it possible for abusive men to change?

It is possible for abusive men to change. Now that you understand that your partner's abusiveness stems from his belief system, however, you can probably appreciate why change is very difficult. We are not talking about his simply needing to manage his anger better or learn better communication skills. Your partner needs to change his deep-seated beliefs about how he relates to you, to his children and to others.

Counseling for abusive men

It is very difficult for people to change their belief structure. It is especially difficult in this situation, because the belief system has been working well for your partner—he has been getting what he wants and has maintained his centrality, superiority and deservedness.

In order to change, your partner has to want to change. He must acknowledge that the problem is abuse and that he is responsible for the abuse. He has to register himself in appropriate counseling and then he has to work hard in his counseling program. He needs to work with a counselor who will challenge his basic ideas and assumptions about relationships and he needs to participate in a counseling group for abusive men. He needs to demonstrate his willingness to be accountable for his behaviour. The more accountability he has, the more likely he is to change and maintain those changes. If he is to change, it will take a long time, but you should notice some significant improvement almost immediately.

Most abusive men resist counseling. They do not want to be challenged. Furthermore, most abusive men do not want others to know about their "bad" behaviour. They want to keep their abuse a secret. Secrecy is part of what keeps the abuse working. If no one knows what your partner is doing to you, his actions have no consequences. It may be hard for you and your partner to imagine him taking part in a counseling program because his abusive behaviour has been a secret for so long. But if your partner is to change, he needs to start being honest about what he is doing.

It is important to keep in mind that abusive men will sometimes use counseling as a tactic to regain control. Think back to the honeymoon phase of the Cycle of Abuse. Many women say that their partner promises to seek counseling during this phase. Some men actually follow through. Attending counseling, rather than just making promises, may be evidence that your partner is committed to change.

If your partner refuses to go or clearly doesn't work hard in his counseling program, it is fair to assume that he will never stop his abusiveness. Even for men who are motivated and work hard, it is difficult to change such fundamental belief structures; it is unlikely your partner will change his on his own.

Anger Management Counseling

Some men who are abusive are referred to anger management programs. However, the problem is not your partner's anger but his underlying belief system. Therefore, it is unlikely that anger management will be beneficial. This can be difficult to understand at first. Your partner's anger is very threatening to you and may seem like the main problem, but it is not. Your partner's belief that he has a right to be central, superior and deserving is the problem. When he feels these beliefs are being challenged, he may respond with anger.

It is also helpful to remember that anger is a tactic your partner uses to maintain power and control over you. His anger is intended to intimidate and silence you. Many women have reported to us that when their partner takes part in an anger management course, they do see some change in their partner's behaviour. For example they may stop hitting, yelling or throwing things. But because the abusive belief system has not been challenged, these men simply develop different tactics to maintain power and control. For example, they may become more emotionally or financially abusive. This dynamic can be very confusing for women. On the surface, it may seem like your partner is "getting better" but in fact he has simply changed his tactics. Ultimately, his intention is to continue to control you.

Couple counseling

You may have wondered if you and your partner should seek counseling together, or perhaps you've already tried this. Based on many women's experience, we advise against couple counseling for three reasons. First, with your partner present, it is unsafe for you to tell the counselor the truth of your relationship. If you do so, you will likely face the negative consequence of your partner's abuse some time after the counseling as he tries to make you pay for what you said.

Second, if you are unable to be honest with the counselor because of your well-grounded fears, you are apt to give the counselor only a partial picture of your relationship. Your partner's behaviour will not look as bad as it is. At the same time, your partner is likely to tell his worst stories about you. As a result, the counselor receives a very inaccurate picture of what's going on and is unhelpful in her or his advice. When abuse is involved, couple counseling is futile at its best and dangerous at its worst.

Third, the problem is your partner's. Couple counseling works when both parties are responsible and both parties want to work towards a solution. However, the abuse is solely your partner's responsibility, and he is the one who has to work at changing his behaviour. After all the abuse has stopped, and you feel safe in expressing yourself, couple counseling may be an important step in establishing a respectful and trusting relationship. This can't happen, though, until you are safe to express yourself.

While your partner is going through counseling, we encourage you to seek a women's group for support. You may find the idea of group counseling with other women who have been abused a little frightening. Perhaps you are influenced by the stereotype of "battered" women that exists in our society. Of all the hundreds of women we've had the pleasure to work with, none of them fit the stereotype—and all of them worried that they wouldn't fit into the group!

Whether your partner is in a counseling program or not, we encourage you to try attending a support group for women who experience abuse. After a few weeks, you'll know whether it is a group that is right for you. It is so much easier to deal with the impact of your partner's abuse with the support of other women who really understand what you have experienced.

What can I expect of my partner?

Sometimes women who have been living with an abusive man for a long time feel that they no longer know what are reasonable expectations of their partner. We don't think this is true. However, in an abusive relationship you can do little to have your expectations met. If you ask for them to be met, you will be accused of nagging. If you insist on them being met, you will be accused of being selfish or controlling. Your partner will become abusive and you will be forced to back down. If you do not back down immediately, the abuse may escalate until you do. After many, many attempts, you have learned that it is futile to express your expectations. You may feel silenced or you may continue to try to express yourself. Either way, your opinions and needs are not valued by your partner.

In our counseling groups, we invite women to brainstorm about what they think are realistic expectations to have in a respectful relationship. We don't ask them to reflect on their own relationship, but rather on the ideas they have about relationships in general. They always come up with a lengthy and perfectly reasonable list. Here is a list from one group:

Reasonable Relationship Expectations

☐	Dedication	☐	Consistent behaviour
☐	Life-long commitment	☐	Humour
☐	Faithfulness	☐	Responsibility
☐	Unconditional love	☐	Sensitivity
☐	Equality	☐	Encouragement

☐ Loyalty	☐ Security (physical, emotional, financial)
☐ Respect	☐ Being listened to
☐ Trust	☐ Caring
☐ Consideration	☐ Being accepted without judgment
☐ Honesty	☐ Shared interests
☐ Shared household and parenting responsibilities	☐ Having decisions trusted
	☐ Concern for my well-being
☐ Tolerance of mistakes	☐ Confidence in the relationship
☐ Support	☐ Attention
☐ Concern for family	☐ Connectedness
☐ Shared decision making	

We hope that the information in this chapter serves to fill in some missing pieces for you as you struggle to make sense of your partner's behaviour. We realize that what you have read may be discouraging for you. Perhaps you didn't realize how differently you and your partner approach your relationship and how fundamental a change he needs to make.

If your partner is really motivated to change, searches out a good counseling program and works hard in that program, it is possible for him to change. You will know if the change is enough to meet your expectations for a respectful and loving relationship.

Some women see, however, that their partners are unwilling to do the hard work that is necessary for a change in their fundamental belief system. If you worry that your partner will not change, it may be hard to know where to find hope. We encourage you to start placing hope in yourself rather than in your partner or the relationship. With the help of supportive people around you, you can start to envision a safer and better life. In chapter 9 we will address how you can search out support for yourself. First, though, let's take a look at how your partner's abuse is affecting your children.

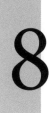

8

What's this doing to my kids?

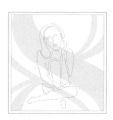

> He says he loves my mom but he lies. He tells my mom to do everything at home. He never gave my mom any money. He hit her; I saw it. I tried to look happy but I wasn't inside. He never played with me—I felt lonely. I feel sad for my dad, he's an idiot. I do not like my dad. When I'm big, I could be Batman and go and kill my dad and throw him in the garbage. I am scared when I have to see my dad, that he will hurt me. ***Boy, aged 6***

How is the abuse affecting my children?

It is very painful to look at how your partner's abuse is affecting your children. You have spent a lot of time wondering about the negative impact on them. You may worry about what your children are learning from your partner's behaviour. You may be concerned that your children will grow up to become abusers or to be abused themselves. All of your concerns are valid. We hope this chapter will help to make some sense of the anxieties you feel for your children.

> I left my husband and got a place for my daughter and myself. I hadn't realized how much my husband's abuse had negatively affected my two-year-old daughter. All of a sudden she would make noise. She would sing and yell and dance around the house. It was wonderful to see. She finally felt safe to be herself. ***Diane***

Your partner's abuse is affecting your children. This will be obvious if your children are witnessing or overhearing the abuse. But even if the abuse only happens when the children are not around, it still affects them negatively because it affects you. The abuse leaves you in poor shape and affects your ability to be the parent you want to be.

Think back to the impact list in chapter 5. Your children will experience impacts similar to yours. Because they do not have the same tools and abilities you have for expressing concerns or accessing resources, they may end up expressing themselves in ways that are hurtful or damaging. Their behaviour may become quite destructive. Alternatively, some children who have witnessed abuse become very "good." They excel in school and never get into trouble. Such children have learned that keeping people with power happy keeps them safe.

If your children have experienced or witnessed abuse, you may be worried about their behaviour. You may wonder if the unacceptable behaviour is because of the abuse or if it is normal childhood behaviour. If, for example, your teenage son suddenly becomes quite rude to you, you may struggle to determine whether he is imitating his father or whether he is just trying to assert normal teenage independence.

First of all, it might be helpful to realize that, on one level, it doesn't matter why your children are behaving inappropriately. If you do not like their behaviour, you need to pay attention to it. Do not disregard it because of the abuse.

Second, it may be helpful to speak with other parents about your children's behaviour. Nurturing friendships with parents of similarly aged children can be helpful. Being a parent is very hard work. We all need to support and help one another. This is especially true if you are not receiving support from your partner. Determine with other parents what is normal behaviour for your children's age group. There is nothing like swapping stories with other parents of adolescents to help you see that your kids are not so bad!

Third, you may want to do some reading. The library can be a great source for resources in parenting. Remember, however, that because your partner is abusive, some advice you will find in books may not apply to your situation.

If you are concerned about how the abuse is affecting your children, you could consider getting them appropriate counseling. Many communities have programs designed for children who have witnessed violence or abuse in their homes. Such counseling will give your children a safe environment to talk about what is going on in their life. Specially trained counselors who are knowledgeable about domestic abuse are a good source of support for both you and your children. You can find out if your community has this form of counseling by calling a transition house or women's shelter.

Why do I feel unable to do what's best for my children?

Often women who are dealing with an abusive partner find themselves severely limited when it comes to providing what is best for their children. For example, women sometimes stay in relationships where they are being abused because they are financially dependent on their partners. They know their partners will fight any attempt to make them pay child support. In such situations women are faced with limited choices. If a woman stays with her partner, the children continue to witness the abuse. If she leaves, she and her children are forced into poverty. Ultimately, the courts can make a father pay child support but the battle is sometimes hard won.

Another dilemma women find themselves in is attempting to protect their children from their father's behaviour. You may have felt pressure either from yourself, from friends or family, or from professionals to remove your children from your partner's abusiveness. However, you may have found that your ability to do so is quite limited. Courts will protect your partner's "right" to have access to his children. Again women find themselves in a no-win situation. If you stay with your partner, you are accused of not shielding your children from abuse. However, if you leave, the courts may give your partner access to the children.

We have not outlined these two difficult scenarios in order to discourage you. We simply hope to identify some of the struggles you may be facing. We also hope to help you to see that the limitations you are experiencing when it comes to providing what is best for your children have more to do with our legal and social systems than they do with your ability as a parent. As a society we need to ensure that fathers pay child support and that children are protected from witnessing or experiencing abuse. Until we do, however, women like you are forced to work within limited parameters. It is possible, with good support and legal advice, to make life for your children safer and better, but it may well be a struggle and you may continue to encounter blocks to doing what you know is best.

Why am I not being the parent I want to be?

Living with an abusive man seriously hampers your ability to be the parent you want to be. Most women worry that they are either "too hard on" or "too lenient with" their children.

Sometimes women find themselves yelling at their children and perhaps even hitting them. Obviously, if you are doing this you are concerned about your behaviour. You know that it is not okay. Your partner's abuse leaves you exhausted and stressed out. Because of this, you probably find that you do not always have the patience that your children require of you. You end up treating your children in ways that are unacceptable.

On the other hand, some women find that they are too lenient with their children. Their children are rude to them or do not behave appropriately. If this is what is happening, you may have realized that you are "easy" on your children in order to compensate for your partner's abuse. You feel that your partner is always giving your children a hard time so you want to give them a break. You may also find that if you try to discipline your children your partner will step in and sabotage your efforts. He either undermines you and tells the children they can disregard what you have said, or he begins to yell at the kids for not "obeying" you.

Why do my children "side" with their father?

Many women are confused by their children's behaviour towards their father. Children will sometimes appear to prefer their father over their mother and defend their father's abusive actions. This is a very painful and confusing experience. We assume that children will position themselves with the safe and dependable parent, but it is precisely because you are safe and dependable that your children can act out against you. Because your partner's behaviour is unpredictable and frightening, your children are less likely to do anything to upset him. You become the parent who can be tested and pushed. The testing of parents is part of normal childhood development, but you are the only parent with whom it is safe to do so.

Your children may also feel that it is necessary to "take sides" in the war your partner is creating. Your partner is the powerful one in your relationship. Aligning themselves with the person who has power is a wise thing for your children to do. It helps keep your children safe.

Living with difficult children is just that—difficult. Try to get as much support for yourself as you can. And take comfort in knowing that your children are so difficult with you because they feel safe with you.

How can I talk to my children about this?

Women struggle with what to say to their children about their partners' abuse. They do not want to sabotage their children's relationship with their father. How can you teach your children about abuse without sounding like you are being unfair to their father?

Remind yourself that if your partner is being abusive he is sabotaging his relationship with his children. His selfishness and abuse hurt you, the children and the stability of your family. These are all consequences of his actions, not yours. If you speak to your children about the abuse, remember that you are only helping your children to understand what your partner is doing. Your partner's behaviour is the problem, and not your speaking about it.

It may also be helpful to separate the abusive behaviour from your partner himself. When talking to your child, try to focus on your partner's behaviour, not on him as a person. Talk about specific situations as abusive or hurtful. Speak to your children only when you are not too upset yourself. Try to put yourself in their situation and think about what is helpful for them to hear from you or talk about with you.

Most research in this area shows that children are far more aware of the abuse than their mothers realize. You may be avoiding this conversation because you think it will be upsetting for your children. However, most children know things are not okay, but do not have the vocabulary to describe what is really going on. If your children know that they can speak to you about the abuse, they will be less afraid. Things will seem a little less out of control. Your children may also let go of the feeling that they are responsible for the abuse or for stopping it.

Will my children grow up to abuse or be abused?

If your children witness your partner's abuse, you are probably concerned about what they are learning. You may worry that your son will grow up to be an abuser or that your daughter will think abuse is "normal" and marry an abusive man. While it is true that your partner's abuse is having a negative effect on your children, it is not true that they are doomed to live in abusive relationships the rest of their lives. You can do a number of things to help your children learn about respectful behaviour.

First, you may consider leaving. Attempting to limit the amount of abuse your children witness is a way to minimize the negative impact your partner is having on them. (We explore this more in chapter 10.)

Second, consider nurturing relationships with people who are positive role models for your children. Do you know men who treat others in respectful, loving ways? Perhaps your children have a grandfather, uncle or family friend who could spend more time with them. Hopefully teachers and coaches will also serve as good role models. We realize your partner may sabotage efforts to provide your children with good role models and isolate you and your children from people outside your home. However, if this is not the case, take some comfort in realizing that your partner is not your children's only model of how to relate to others.

Third, talk to your children about abusive and respectful behaviour. As much as possible, teach your children the vocabulary necessary to describe what is acceptable and appropriate versus disrespectful and abusive. If it is difficult to talk about your partner's behaviour, use others as material for discussion. Talk about behaviour you see in the mall or on television. If some behaviour is abusive, call it that. If you experience kind and respectful behaviour, comment on it. Try to talk about all the different kinds of abuse. Be sure that your children know about verbal and emotional abuse and not just physical abuse. If you are not living with your partner, and if your children are old enough, you may be able to draw a Power and Control Wheel with them. Have your children identify the different types of abuse they have witnessed or experienced. If you give your children the vocabulary to understand abusive behaviour, they are then able to draw their own conclusions about their father's behaviour.

Remember that people who were raised in abusive homes can choose to live in a different way as adults. If you give your children the vocabulary they need for understanding abuse and its effects on others, you will help them to choose to live free of abuse.

In this chapter, we have tried to address the anxieties you have when it comes to your children. Because of your partner's abuse, you are forced to carry a lot of responsibility. You have lots of evidence to suggest that your partner will not put the physical and emotional needs of his children before his own needs. This leaves you to look out for their interests. As well, you know from experience that there are limits put on you when it comes to doing what is best for your children; limits imposed by your partner, his abusive behaviour, or the courts. Nevertheless, we hope that through this chapter we have affirmed you in what you are already doing for your children as well as giving you some ideas of things you might do in the future to support them and to get support for them from the community. However, it is not only your children who need and deserve support right now. You do too. Our next chapter will look at ways to get the help you need.

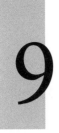

9

Am I getting the support I need?

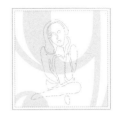

> I needed to tell someone. I needed support from people who would be concerned for my safety and well-being. A friend referred me to a counseling agency. I entered a support group for women. The first few weeks of group counseling were wonderful for me. I began to understand how so much of Peter's behaviour towards me was abusive. I discovered that I didn't deserve the treatment I received. I discovered I was not crazy. And I discovered I was not alone. **Marion**

How do I know if I'm getting the right support?

This book has taken you through a difficult journey, exploring your relationship from the perspective of inequality and abuse. At this point, we'd like to invite you to think about additional sources of support. Your partner's abuse has far-reaching implications for you and has affected many aspects of your life. Because his abuse has likely affected you mentally, emotionally, physically, spiritually and financially, you may need to draw on a range of supportive services in order to deal with the impact of the abuse. You need to know how to access resources such as the police, legal services, health services, social services and appropriate counseling.

While there are many good services to support women who have experienced abuse, unfortunately not all sources of support are helpful. Sometimes women are given dangerous advice (for example, therapists may tell women to stand up to their partners). Sometimes police don't show up when they're called, and sometimes social service workers treat women disrespectfully.

Listed below are some potential sources of support. Some of these sources may not be relevant for you, while you may already significantly rely on others. Start by evaluating the support you have right now.

Here are some criteria for evaluating a potential source of support:

1. Do they believe me 100 percent of the time?

2. Are they concerned about my emotional and physical well-being more than they are concerned about my partner or the relationship?

3. Are they trustworthy? Do I know that they will respect the confidentiality of what I tell them?

4. Do they emphasize my strengths and affirm me?

5. Are they dependable? Can I rely on them to be reasonably available when I need them?

Use these criteria, along with your own ideas about good support, to evaluate your current situation. Place a check mark in the box beside the person or institution who is a source of support for you. Leave the box blank if you have had no contact with this person or institution. Place an "X" in the box if your experience with this person or institution has been negative.

Potential Sources of Support

☐ Doctor

☐ Lawyer

☐ Police

☐ Employment (boss/co-workers)

☐ Counselors for you or for your children

☐ Employment training

☐ Child care

☐ Children's school

☐ Group counseling

☐ Recreation centre, social club, hobby club

☐ Friends

☐ Family

☐ Social services/social worker

☐ Transition house

☐ Food bank

☐ Church/faith community

☐ Spiritual leader

☐ _____

_____

☐ _____

_____

☐ _____

_____

What is my Circle of Support?

Now let's think a little bit more about your responses. Look at the diagram below.

Circle of Support

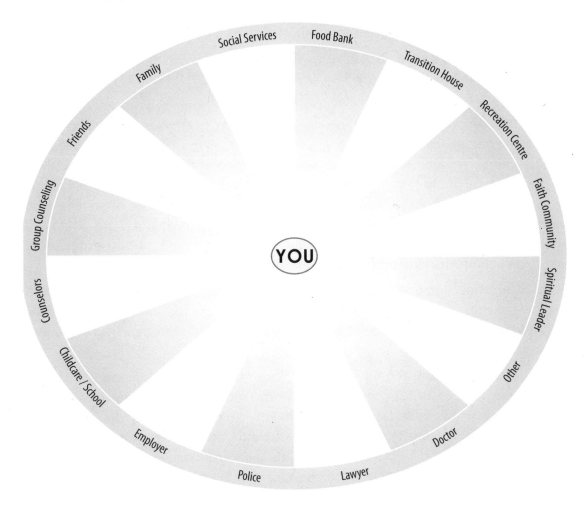

For each category, describe how or why this person or institution is helpful or unhelpful to you. For example, one woman might report that her doctor does not listen well and jumps in too quickly with easy solutions. Another woman may find her doctor to be very supportive, a good listener and genuinely concerned about her mental and physical well-being. As you think about these people and places, you may discover that some of them are supportive sometimes, but not at other times. When you are finished, put a star beside those persons or institutions who consistently give you good and dependable support.

What are the barriers to my getting support?

Many women find barriers that block them from good support. Some of these barriers come from limits imposed by their partner. If a woman's partner limits her access to the phone, car or money, it is difficult to access some services. Some women can't afford to speak to a lawyer or can't get the car to visit a friend. Abusive men also use threats to try to limit their partner's access to services, such as the police.

Some services are difficult to access. Women may face long waiting lists for employment training or counseling for their children. Sometimes they do not qualify for the service that they need (e.g., legal aid).

Some of the barriers to accessing these services have to do with women's well-founded fears. For example, thinking about going to a transition house or women's shelter for the first time is very frightening. Everyone is anxious when dealing with the unknown. You may also be afraid that you don't "fit the stereotype" and therefore don't qualify for the service. For example, women without broken bones or bruises often think they do not qualify for counseling for "battered" women. Furthermore, if you are exhausted because of the abuse, embarrassed by your situation or have had bad experiences with some institutions in the past, you are less likely to reach out for help.

As you think about some of the barriers that keep you from accessing what might be helpful resources for you, add these barriers under the appropriate headings on the diagram. Some barriers, such as lack of money or personal fears, may show up under a number of headings.

Now look at the diagram you have created. Take note of how many stars you have—dependable sources of support. Also note how many barriers to services or bad experiences you have had. Does it seem that you are receiving good support from a variety of important sources? If you are, that is wonderful. This, however, would be unusual. Women often find only a few sources of support, and some institutions or individuals who attempt to be supportive turn out to be disappointing. Here are some examples:

Yan Wha

Yan Wha finally gets up the courage to call the police after one of her husband's physical assaults. When the police question her, she feels she's being interrogated. When she has no physical evidence to show them, they grow skeptical. She asks them to remove her husband from the home. After speaking with him, however, they clearly accept his version of the story and do not remove him.

The police should have believed Yan Wha and been concerned for her safety. They should have either removed her partner or taken her to a safe place.

Beth

After a night of relentless emotional abuse, Beth goes to see her pastor. For the first time, she really reveals how terrible her family situation is for her. Her pastor seems genuinely concerned and she finds herself telling him more than she intended. The pastor promises to be helpful to Beth and says a prayer with her. Beth leaves the office feeling better. She is shocked, however, when her husband comes home early from work, in a rage. The pastor had stopped by his work and confronted him about his behaviour in the marriage.

Although Beth did not think to state her need for confidentiality, her pastor should have assumed it. Although her pastor's actions were well-intentioned, they put Beth at risk.

Sarah

Sarah is living with her husband and is beginning to consider a separation. She decides to see a counselor for support and for help in sorting through her complex situation. She goes to a counselor who has been highly recommended by a friend. The counselor tells her that he would like to see her and her husband together. What follows is a series of marriage counseling sessions with the goal of mending the relationship. Sarah is given a lot of advice for dealing with the conflict and anger in her relationship. The therapist tells Sarah that relationship conflict is normal and that it is important for her to hear her partner's anger without retreating. The counselor suggests that her inability to deal with her partner's anger stems from her father's anger.

Sarah knows from experience that asserting herself puts her at risk of a verbal or physical assault from her partner. Furthermore, the counselor's focus on Sarah as the one with "the problem" does not affirm or strengthen her. Finally, the suggestion that the problem is anger rather than abuse makes the impact of abuse invisible.

These examples are not intended to discourage you but to make one simple point. If you have not received the support you need, it is not your fault. It can be difficult to find good support. It may be helpful to broaden your sources of support, although this can be difficult. You know that it can be risky to tell someone about your situation. You don't know if they will believe you and you may wonder if they are dependable and trustworthy.

Unfortunately, you need to be a wise consumer when it comes to support. If a salesperson at your local department store were rude to you, you would likely shop elsewhere next time. Similarly, if someone who is supposed to be supporting you is not, you need to look elsewhere.

We realize how difficult this is. It is much more difficult to change your doctor or your faith community than it is to change shopping patterns. However, it will ultimately be more helpful to you if you're able to find some true support for yourself. We also realize that we are sometimes stuck with people or institutions. For example, your boss may be completely unsympathetic to your situation but you may be in no position to change jobs. Of course, you also have no control over who makes up your family. You can't trade your parents or siblings for ones that might be more understanding or supportive. If you realize how supportive or unsupportive these non-negotiable people are, you can then be realistic about the role they will play in your life at this time. If your boss is unsupportive, don't look to him or her for support. Perhaps a co-worker will provide better support. If your siblings continue to be critical of you, you may choose to spend less time with them, at least for now. You are in a critical and difficult time in your life. Try not to waste your limited energy on people who are unable or unwilling to support you.

Although it is difficult to find good support, it is certainly not impossible. Often the best source for information is your local transition house or women's shelter. You do not need to actually stay at one of these facilities in order to use their services. You can call them for suggestions about counseling programs, lawyers and dealing with social services. If you do not know the phone number of your closest shelter or transition house, consider calling the crisis line in the front of your local phone book and ask them for the phone number. The internet can also be a good source for information. However, you may want to consider using a computer that your partner does not have access to, such as one in a public library.

You may find that the services you seek are described as being for "battered women." It is important to know that you do not need to have been physically assaulted to take advantage of these services. Professionals who work in this field recognize that abuse takes many forms.

Finding an appropriate form of counseling for yourself can be a very helpful step towards getting the support you need and deserve. You can find out if there is a support group for abused women in your community by calling a transition house, a women's resource centre or the YWCA. Connecting with women who have had similar experiences can be an invaluable resource for you.

Sometimes women who have experienced abuse also struggle with substance abuse or mental health issues. If this is true for you, you may experience even more barriers to finding good support. For example, some programs tell women that they must "deal with their addiction" before they can access services. As we found in chapter 4, there is a connection between living through the trauma of abuse and developing substance use or mental illness. Many women who have experienced mental health problems such as depression or anxiety report that these conditions were a result of the abuse they experienced. As one woman said, "Some people call it mental ill health. I call it symptoms of abuse." If you had mental health challenges before your relationship began, you may have noticed that these problems have worsened because of the abuse.

Similarly, there is a link between woman abuse and substance use. Perhaps you drink or use substances to numb the pain of the abuse or escape the constant fear and dread associated with the relationship. An abusive partner may also coerce or force you to use substances with him, and this might be safer for you than resisting. Whatever your reasons, it is important to know that you are coping the best you can.

Unfortunately, not all service providers have made this connection, which makes services less accessible for you. You may be afraid to tell someone about your struggles with substances or mental ill health because you fear that your children will be taken away from you. You may also have been made to feel ashamed for using street or prescription drugs to cope. Take heart. It may take some work to find an organization or person that sees the links between substance use, mental ill health and experiences of abuse.

Women often want to gather legal information in order to protect themselves and their children should they decide to leave at some point. Friends or family members may give you advice, but remember the law is very complicated. Well-meaning people sometimes give faulty information. As well, your partner may have intimidated you with legal threats that you will want to check out with an expert. It is very important for you to know your legal rights, especially when children are involved. You can access legal information by calling Legal Aid or Legal Services in your phone book.

How can I plan ahead?

It may be difficult to plan for the future. Part of the struggle may be that your partner's abuse leaves you exhausted and off-balance. Because of this, it may be difficult to do more than just get through the day. For some women, the physical, financial or social threats their partner throws at them keep them from making plans for the future. We recognize all of these barriers and understand what a paralyzing effect they may have on you.

We would, however, encourage you to do as much thinking about the future as you are able. It may be difficult right now to contemplate needing to leave your home, but this need may arise at some point. It is much more difficult to think about what you should do when you are in the middle of the crisis than if you have a plan in place ahead of time. Remind yourself that just because you have a plan doesn't mean you have to use it. For example, you can say to yourself, "If I had to leave, this is where I would go."

You may also be thinking about separating from your partner permanently. Often this seems completely overwhelming. Working on a long-term plan for leaving can break a seemingly overwhelming problem into smaller, attainable steps. Start by gathering resources and information for yourself.

For example, going to a lawyer and seeking advice about protecting your children and your financial security can be an important step. It would be wise not to tell your partner if you see a lawyer. Even though it may seem deceptive to keep this information from him, remember that your partner's belief structure permits him to put his needs and desires before yours or your children's (see chapter 7). In the event of a separation, his main concern will be his own well-being. Unfortunately, that leaves only you to be concerned about yourself and your children. Consulting a lawyer is an important step in protecting yourself and them.

Every woman is in a unique situation and has different things to consider as she thinks about her future. For this reason we have included some concrete ideas about planning in different situations. Please look at these ideas and decide what fits your experience.

If you are living with your partner

► Decide where you will go if you have to leave home, even if you don't think you will have to. Where would you go if your first choice didn't work out?

► Know how to exit safely. What doors, windows, elevators, stairwells or fire escapes would you use?

► Keep your purse and car keys in a place where you can get to them if you have to leave quickly.

► Tell your neighbours about your concerns and ask that they call the police if they hear suspicious noises coming from your house.

► Teach your children to use the phone to contact the police and fire department.

- Use a code word with your children or friends so they can call for help.

- When you expect that there is going to be an argument, avoid the bathroom, garage, kitchen and other areas near weapons, or rooms without access to an outside door.

- Use your judgment and intuition. If the situation is very serious, you may decide to give your partner what he wants to calm him down. Do what you need to do to protect yourself until you are out of danger.

If you are thinking about leaving

- Consider opening up a savings account for yourself.

- Consider opening your own post office box.

- Consider opening a floating voice mail box. Do not give your partner the phone number.

- Try to find employment if you are unemployed.

- Research resources in your community (e.g., food bank).

- Speak to the staff at a transition house.

- Discover which friends will support and help you.

- Look at places to rent.

- Keep copies of important documents, keys, clothes and money with a friend or family member.

- Keep numbers of important resources with you or memorize these numbers.

- Explore employment courses through local colleges.

If you or your partner has left

- Change the locks on doors and replace wooden doors with metal doors. Install additional locks, window bars or poles to wedge against doors.

- Get an unlisted phone number and call screening.

- Teach your children how to use the telephone to make a collect call to you in the event your partner takes the children.

- Tell people who take care of your children who can pick them up and that your partner is not permitted to do so.

- Inform neighbours and friends that your partner no longer resides with you and that they should call the police if he is seen near your home.

- ▶ Plan ahead for what you can do if you feel down and ready to return to a potentially abusive situation.

- ▶ Find friends or family members you can call for support.

- ▶ Develop a plan that best protects your safety for when and/or if you have to communicate with your partner in person or by telephone.

This chapter has listed a lot of practical suggestions, which we hope will help you. It may be overwhelming to think about all you could do to gather support or to plan for the future. Try not to get overwhelmed by taking on too much at once. Instead, ask yourself if there is one thing you could do to get more support for yourself or to plan for the future. For example, one woman realized she needed to get out of her car loan and buy a less expensive car if she was ever to be financially independent of her partner. She hadn't decided yet if she was going to separate from her partner, but she wanted to be debt-free regardless. Putting her car up for sale was an attainable step that made it more possible to leave her partner. It did not mean, however, that she had to leave him.

Women sometimes find there are things they can do that will give them more support or open up some options for them without forcing a decision about staying or leaving. Each little step you make is very significant. Some of the steps you make do not seem visible. They have to do with how you are thinking and feeling rather than what you are doing. However, women who have worked through this process tell us that some of these small steps, such as changing how they thought about themselves, made a big difference. By beginning to realize that you are in a very difficult situation and deserve some affirmation and support, you are taking a very significant step.

We hope this chapter has given you some helpful ideas about what you can do to find support during this difficult time. In our next chapter, we will discuss the many factors you need to consider when deciding to leave, or to stay with, your abusive partner.

10

Should I leave him?

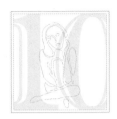

I thought a lot about leaving but I was torn. I still loved Michael, but his treatment of me was intolerable. I also felt I couldn't deal with the terrible embarrassment of a separation. Perhaps even more important, I was afraid to be alone. One of the impacts of Michael's abuse was that I thought poorly of myself. I thought that no other man would want to be with me. It felt like Michael was my only chance for marriage and family. I didn't want to stay in an abusive relationship, but if I left I might be alone for the rest of my life. The whole dilemma seemed overwhelming. *Kate*

Through the process of reading this book, you have done some hard work in order to evaluate your relationship. You have explored the different ways your partner has abused you and the impact that abuse has had on you and your children. A careful examination of your partner's abuse has perhaps made you wonder if you should leave him. This is a difficult and painful question to ask. It brings to the surface a myriad of emotional and practical concerns. In this chapter, we will explore this very complex question.

Staying or leaving?

We have noticed, and you probably have too, that if you confide in anyone about your partner, the first reaction is "Why are you still with him?" You may also have your own questions about this. If you've left the relationship, you may wonder why you stayed as long as you did.

Our society offers only two possibilities regarding relationships—staying or leaving. Either you're with your partner or you've left him. This seems to apply to all relationships, not just abusive ones. However, when women are in an abusive relationship, people seem to feel more justified in offering the simple (and naive) solution of leaving. Perhaps you yourself wonder why you remain with a partner who is not respectful.

If you are still working on a relationship with your partner—whether you are living together or separately—it might be helpful to list the reasons that you are still committed to your relationship. If you have left your partner, think back to the reasons why you stayed for the time that you did.

My Reasons for Staying

_____

_____

_____

_____

_____

_____

Women have shared with us the following reasons for staying, some of which may be on your list:

▶ I still love him!

▶ I don't want to be alone.

▶ I take my marriage vows very seriously.

▶ I want to get back what we once had.

▶ I still have dreams and hope for the future.

▶ I feel embarrassed about being abused.

▶ I'm worried about the effects of divorce on the children.

▶ I share financial commitments with my partner.

▶ I don't know if financially and emotionally I can manage on my own.

▶ I'm worried that single parenting will be too hard.

- ▶ I'm feeling too exhausted or overwhelmed to make a big decision.
- ▶ I hold strong values and ideas about marriage and commitment.
- ▶ I feel strongly identified as a couple with friends, family and my community.
- ▶ I'm afraid of disappointing family.
- ▶ I want the children to have a father.
- ▶ I feel sorry for him.
- ▶ I don't want to lose my home.
- ▶ He's never physically abused me.
- ▶ At least he doesn't drink.
- ▶ He's threatened to kill himself.
- ▶ He's in counseling. I'm waiting to see if he changes.
- ▶ He has some redeeming qualities to which I am holding on.
- ▶ He has threatened to hurt me if I leave with the children.
- ▶ He has threatened to get custody of the children if I leave.

Generally, women say that they want the abuse to end, not the relationship. Even if you have separated in order to gain some safety, you may wish to continue to work with your partner on creating a safe and positive relationship.

We recognize that living separately—whether that is establishing your own home, staying with friends or family, or going to a transition house for awhile—doesn't necessarily mean you want to or intend to end the relationship. It means that you are attempting to establish expectations for a respectful and mutual relationship.

You are doing what you can to make sense of this relationship for yourself. When you're ready, you'll make a decision that is right for you.

Why is it hard even to think about leaving?

When evaluating why you stay in your relationship, it may be helpful to realize how the impact of the abuse plays a role in keeping you in the relationship. Abuse from an intimate partner often leaves a woman feeling exhausted, overwhelmed and confused. Deciding to leave your partner is no doubt one of the hardest decisions you will ever make. It is hard to make such a difficult decision when you feel paralyzed by all the abuse. Women describe a lengthy and painful process in making the decision to leave an abusive partner. They don't wake up one morning and say to themselves "my partner is abusive and I need to leave." Women who do leave often take lots of time to think about and plan ahead for a separation.

It may also be helpful to remind yourself that any woman would find it very difficult and stressful to leave the person she thought she had committed to for life. Even if your partner were not abusive, it would be overwhelming to deal with all the things related to a separation (e.g., moving house, effects on your children, reactions of family and friends, embarrassment, etc.). When you add to it the exhaustion, frayed nerves and fear that come from living with an abusive man, it may seem almost impossible.

Shouldn't I stay while my partner is in counseling?

Sometimes women feel that they need to stand by their partners if they seek counseling. Women do this out of a sense of wanting to give their partners a "fair" chance. First of all, you probably don't need to worry about being "fair." You have likely given your partner many, many chances to change. Second, there is no reason why you can't live apart while your partner is in counseling and then assess at the end of his program if he has changed enough for you to want to try the relationship again. In fact, your partner may be more motivated if he realizes that the relationship is at stake if he doesn't change. In our experience, abusive men won't even attempt to change unless they believe they have something significant to lose.

Your partner may try to convince you that he's changed "enough" and that you should be grateful. We hope you'll be able to evaluate your partner's changes in terms of your own expectations. Only you can decide whether the changes your partner has made make you feel safe and respected in your relationship. Trust yourself.

Why is my partner still abusive even though I've left him?

Unfortunately, your partner may continue the Cycle of Abuse whether you are with him or not. Let's look at Elaine's story.

Elaine

Elaine has left her partner and is hiding from him at a co-worker's house. She has wisely chosen to stay with someone her husband doesn't know. He initially tries to find her by using honeymoon behaviour on her family and friends. He expresses great concern for Elaine to her parents and insists that he is willing to cooperate in whatever ways are necessary to overcome their problems. He says similar things to the rest of her family. When it becomes clear that Elaine's family is not willing to betray her, her partner moves on to tension-building behaviour, pestering and harassing her family with phone calls. Finally he explodes, smashing the windshield of her sister's car.

There seem to be many ways for an abusive man to continue the Cycle even if you are not with him. For example, he may use the court system, threatening to sue for custody of your children or refusing to cooperate in releasing fifty percent of the assets from the marriage. Because abusive men continue the Cycle, women have to continue to be on guard.

This can be discouraging. You would like to think that once you have left your partner he will no longer have the ability to hurt you. This is not always the case. Many women have found, however, that once they are no longer living with their partners and are no longer exposed to the constant abuse, the impact of the abuse begins to lessen. Living with abuse is exhausting and leaves you feeling that you can't cope. Most women feel safer and stronger when there is some distance between themselves and their partners.

How will leaving affect my children?

Women often feel trapped in a no-win situation when they think about how leaving will affect their children. If you are currently living with your partner, you worry about the abuse your children are witnessing or experiencing. Perhaps you have been criticized by others for "letting" your children be exposed to this. Alternatively, if you have decided to separate from your partner, you will worry about depriving your children of a father and may be criticized by others for this. The whole question of staying or leaving becomes even more complicated when children are involved. No matter what you do, you may feel guilty and will likely experience criticism from others.

There is another way to look at your situation. It may be helpful to realize that you are not responsible for providing your children with a good father; only your partner has this ability. Only he has control over whether he is a good father or not.

If your partner is abusing the children, or abusing you in front of the children, you may choose to leave for the sake of your children's emotional and physical well-being. Such a move would serve to protect your children but it does not alter whether your partner is a good father or not. Furthermore, your ability to keep your children safe may be limited if your partner is threatening to sue for custody of the children or is stalking you or the children.

If you keep reminding yourself that only your partner can choose to be a good father, your questions about staying or leaving may change. Remember, your partner can choose to be a good father whether you live with him or not. The two are not tied to each other, as the following story illustrates.

Susan and Ted

Ted had been abusive to Susan for many years. Ted began attending a group for abusive men and Susan went to a support group for women. Ted's behaviour began to improve but Susan realized that she really wanted and needed to live apart from him, at least for a while. Ted continued to attend his group and began behaving in ways that were thoughtful and respectful of Susan and their two children. Over time Susan realized that she no longer wanted to live with Ted but was very interested in him being a good father to their children. Because Ted had stopped being abusive and was being respectful to Susan, the two of them worked out a reasonable custody agreement. The children now spend time with their father, who treats both them and their mother in respectful ways.

This story shows that a man can choose to be a good father whether he lives with his children or not. The choice is his. Also remember that part of being a good father is treating you well.

Am I ready to be a single parent?

You may worry about leaving your partner and trying to be a parent on your own. Being a single parent is extremely difficult. You may be concerned not only about the emotional pressures of single parenting but also about the financial and social pressures.

If you are living with your partner, it might be helpful to analyze how difficult your current situation is. You may already be doing most of the parenting work. Pause for a moment and think this through. Try listing what you do to care for the children and what he does. Remember to record such things as housework, cooking, shopping, laundry, doctor's appointments, soccer games, trips to the library and household scheduling.

Am I Ready to be a Single Parent?

Me: **Him:**

_____   _____

_____   _____

_____   _____

_____   _____

_____   _____

_____   _____

_____   _____

_____   _____

In looking at your two lists, you may realize that your partner is not currently contributing very much to your children's well-being. If this is the case, it may be easier to think about managing on your own with your children. On the other hand, you may also realize that your partner offers some very important and valuable things to your children. If this is the case, remember Ted and Susan's story: living apart from your partner does not negate his ability to be a good parent.

It is also helpful to remember that dealing with an abusive partner is exhausting. You may feel at the end of your rope and feel you couldn't possibly survive as a single parent. But remember that you are exhausted because of your partner's abuse. If you weren't so tired and stressed out from the abuse, the chores of parenting would not seem so overwhelming. This can be difficult to see when you are living with the abuse or dealing with it on an ongoing basis.

What if I don't want my children to see their father?

Common belief says that children should maintain contact with their father, but this is not always the case. Rather than holding on to this generalization, think about your particular situation. If your partner abuses your children or his abuse of you affects them negatively, then you have good reason to want to limit his contact. You are being a good mother and are attempting to protect your children from abuse.

You may not have the final say on whether your partner will have access to your children. Courts are hesitant to limit a father's access to his children. You may find yourself fighting for limited or no access and having few allies. You may be made to feel selfish or hateful. If this is the case, re-examine your motives. If your concern is for the welfare of your children, do not feel bad. Remember, you know your children and your family situation better than anyone else; you are the expert on the welfare of your children.

If you share children with your abusive partner, you are facing a very difficult and painful reality. Like it or not, you have a link with your partner that will last at least until your children are grown. Your partner may try to maintain control over you through your children. Fighting for custody or failing to provide support payments is a powerful way to hurt you and maintain power over you.

Perhaps the biggest fear most women hold is that of losing their children. They are afraid that they will either lose custody of their children or lose their children's respect and love. In working with women, we have witnessed that, when it comes to parenting, the long term matters. Your partner may try to win your children's favour by buying expensive gifts. He may tell lies about you that your children believe for awhile. These are painful experiences. But your partner will not be a consistently "good" parent. You can be a source of stability for your children. You can be dependable, predictable, loving, honest and respectful. For most children, this is what matters in the long run.

We hope this chapter has addressed some of the questions you have as you consider whether or not to leave your partner. We also hope we have honoured how truly painful the question is. We know that it is never an easy decision. It is not our intention to convince you to leave. We believe that you are in the best position to make that decision for yourself. None of us can make that judgment for each other. You know what is best for you—and what is safest.

11

How do I heal from the abuse?

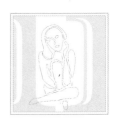

For several days I had been feeling really strong and happy. I had thought very little about my ex-partner. But then I took our daughter to the pool for a swim. I saw all of those moms and dads together with their kids, and sadness flooded over me. I saw in those families what I had always wanted for my daughter and me. It feels discouraging. How much longer am I going to feel all of this pain? When am I going to feel like I'm really getting on with my life? **Lynn**

Why does this hurt so much?

Each woman's journey to wholeness, after the devastating experience of abuse, is unique, yet there are some important similarities. The healing process tends to involve periods of intense grief and sadness as well as periods of rebuilding and hope. These two experiences may feel unrelated, but for us, they are the two sides of a coin; they go together. This will become clearer as you read this chapter; let's begin by talking about the grieving part of the healing process.

Whether or not you have left your partner, you may find yourself overwhelmed with feelings of sadness, loss and grief. Your life is not the way you had dreamed it would be, and if you have children, many of your hopes and dreams for them may not be met either. Added to your many and complex emotions is the fact that you may feel alone in your pain. You may be keeping many of your feelings to yourself because your friends and family don't understand what you are going through, and they can't offer the support you need and deserve.

A woman leaving, or considering leaving, an abusive partner moves through a journey of grief that can be complex and lengthy. First of all, her loss may not be socially recognized. In our society, we are given permission to grieve only certain types of losses. For example, the death of a parent, child or spouse is deemed a significant loss, and people will offer support. For these losses, funerals are held, flowers are sent and companies give their employees days off work. However, other types of losses go largely unrecognized by our communities.

For the most part, people do not recognize separation or divorce in terms of significant loss. They assume that when a marriage "doesn't work" both parties choose to separate. Even if it is recognized as a painful process, society does not create much opportunity for grieving. From our perspective, separation and divorce are excruciating. At the end of a relationship, you may experience many of the same losses as someone whose partner has died. For example, you may feel that:

▶ you have lost the person you once loved and imagined to be a life partner;

▶ you have lost what you envisioned your relationship or family would look like;

▶ you have lost the "dream" of what your life would be like.

On top of this, because your partner is abusive, your grieving process may be even more complex, and there may be added dimensions to your loss. For example, women usually lose contact with their in-laws (who are sometimes as dear to them as their own blood relatives). They are also likely to lose former friends who believe their ex-partners' lies. Furthermore, because financial abuse is often present, there are huge financial impacts such as losing a home or falling into debt. Janette's story illustrates some of these additional complexities, and it highlights similarities and differences between different endings to two different relationships.

Janette

I lost my first husband to kidney failure. It was horrible. He was sick for a long time before he finally died, and when he was finally gone, I was devastated. My family and church community were wonderful, however. I was allowed to be an emotional wreck. I cried a lot. People took my kids so I could have time to myself. Friends were always bringing over food – our fridge was full of home-cooked meals, cookies and cakes. Losing my husband this way was really awful, but my community saw me through it, and after many months, the pain and loss I felt began to lift.

My second marriage, in contrast, ended because my husband was abusive. Compared to the death of my first husband, the grief was just as bad, but it was much more complicated. I was very confused for a long time, and it was all very messy. Before I left for good, I went back to my husband many times, so there was no clear break. My children (now grown) became very judgemental of me. They wanted me out of the relationship and could not understand why I kept going back. I loved my husband. I wanted the relationship to work out. I wanted the abuse to end, not the relationship.

When I finally decided the relationship was over, I was devastated, but no one, except the women in my support group, could understand my grief. Some people thought I should have left my husband long ago and thought I should "just be happy to be out." Others judged me for ending my marriage and had no sympathy for my painfully difficult decision.

My two experiences of grief were so entirely different. With the death of my second marriage I was expected to swallow my pain. There was no formal recognition of my loss (something that a funeral provides), and no one brought casseroles or homemade cookies.

As Janette's story illustrates, sometimes a woman's grief is minimized, and her loss is not recognized. People say things like "she chose to leave," or "he was so terrible, she should be glad to be out." Other times, women are judged for choosing to end a relationship and consequently don't get the support that they need. Judgements may include "he never hit her," "he didn't cheat on her," or "surely, it wasn't that bad."

Remember that if you are contemplating leaving your partner, or have already done so, you are probably going through one of the most painful periods of your life. Are you receiving the support and understanding that you need considering all of your losses?

A woman in your situation has many things to grieve. Here is a list of some things that women say about their grief:

- ▶ "I grieve the loss of who I thought my husband was."
- ▶ "I no longer trust the person I thought I could trust the most."
- ▶ "I grieve the death of my hopes and dreams."
- ▶ "My life is not at all how I wanted it to be."
- ▶ "My family, as I knew it, is gone."
- ▶ "I only have my children 50% of the time."
- ▶ "I lost the opportunity to be a 'stay at home mom'. I have to work."
- ▶ "My children turned against me."
- ▶ "I lost my home and my garden."
- ▶ "I lost most of my friends and my faith community."

- "I've lost social status." (I feel labelled – "divorced," "single mom," "broken home.")
- "I lost all sense of financial security."
- "I feel like I've lost the best years of my life."
- "I'm feeling the loss of opportunities (education, career etc.)"
- "I lost everything!"

If your relationship has ended or is ending, your losses are enormous. The grief and pain you feel may seem too much to bear at times, and if you are like most women in your situation, your community is not likely to recognize your suffering. You may not even recognize all of your own losses.

Why is it hard to grieve?

We know that grief can be a lengthy and painful process that follows any significant loss. It is normal for us to grieve all sorts of things such as the loss of an enjoyable job or a loss of health. Likewise, the end of any significant relationship requires time to grieve. However, there are many reasons why women leaving abusive relationships may be prevented from expressing their grief.

Sometimes women feel frozen in their grief for a time. That is, they have to postpone their grieving for one or several reasons. We know that just because a woman leaves, it does not mean that the abuse ends. So, you may be frozen in your grief in order to stay emotionally tough and fight to protect yourself, your children or your financial security. In this case, the person whose loss you are grieving continues to hurt you; you may find yourself swinging from extreme sadness to extreme anger with each new assault from your ex-partner.

In the following example, Frances describes how she feels, "I'm just trying to survive... I can't tend to my wounds because I am still in the battle."

> When I left my relationship, my partner immediately began legal action against me. He tried to prove in court that I was an unfit parent. I had to fight with everything that I had to protect my infant son. In the midst of such a momentous battle, there was no time to grieve that my marriage was over. I was angry, and I was scared, but it wasn't until the court process was over that I could feel sad for all of my losses. (Happily, I was successful in court and my ex-partner's claims were exposed as lies.) **Frances**

You may also be frozen in grief because you are overwhelmed with practical concerns. You may have to find a new home, get a job or find childcare. These things would be challenging under any circumstances, but after an abusive relationship it is even more difficult. Fear, fatigue, lack of support, financial stress and poor health are just some of the things that may be contributing to your sense of being overwhelmed.

Our society's expectations in such a situation are quite unrealistic. Would we expect a hostage victim, after years of captivity, to immediately go and find a job, rent a new home, buy a car, and fill the cupboards with groceries? Probably not. We would provide such a person with time to heal; we would recognize the terrible emotional cost of the experience and allow for recovery. Similarly, what a woman leaving abuse really needs is time to heal, grieve, and gather her strength, but that is not usually what she gets. Most women feel like all they are doing is "surviving" for the first year or so after separation. They don't have the time or emotional energy to tally all of their losses. The daily demands of life leave little space for personal reflection. And if they have children, they may find themselves focused more on the children's emotional needs than on their own.

Then, sometimes a long time after the separation, feelings of sadness sweep over them, often unexpectedly. Suddenly they can feel quite overwhelmed by their losses. Unfortunately, by this time some family and friends think that they should be "over it."

A further complication to the grieving process in situations of abuse is that the losses often come over a series of years or even decades.

> The death of my marriage was gradual, over many years. Mark's hateful behaviour was like a cancer that gradually killed my love for him. Mark didn't die, but my love for him sure did. It was a slow and painful process, and I was aware of grieving a lot while I was still with him. I would think things like 'well, I guess this is all that I can expect' and feel very sad that my marriage was not what I wanted it to be. **Jody**

In some ways, Jody's description of her grief is like that of a person who loses a loved one to a disease like Alzheimer's. It is gradual, slow and very painful.

Why do I have such mixed emotions about the end of my relationship?

In our experience, most women find the first few years after separation to be a roller coaster of emotions. Sometimes they feel all of the losses of the relationship while other times they are relieved and happy to have left. As life evolves, many women begin to feel excited and even joyful in their new found freedom and independence.

It is normal to have a diverse mixture of emotions. In fact, moving through various thoughts and feelings is a key component to healing from the abuse you have experienced.

Diagram 11.1   The Healing Process

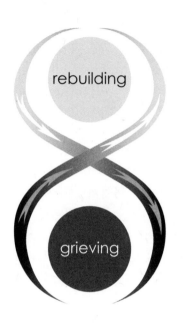

Here is a diagram that illustrates what the healing process may look like for you:

The top part of the figure, titled Rebuilding, is the part of the healing process when you are moving forward and feeling more hopeful about your future. The abuse has taken so much away from you, and here you are rebuilding that which your partner tore down. Here are some things that women tell us they experience during these times.

Check off the emotions that fit for you.

Rebuilding Emotions

☐ I feel hopeful

☐ I feel strong

☐ I feel at peace

☐ I feel safe (or safer)

☐ I feel "normal"

☐ I feel relief

☐ I feel energized

☐ I feel euphoric at times

☐ I experience joy

☐ I am able to make long-term decisions

☐ I am optimistic

☐ I have more clarity

☐ I see possibilities

☐ I feel more in control

☐ I feel more confident

☐ I trust myself

☐ I trust my instincts

☐ I like myself

- ☐ I feel cheerful
- ☐ I feel affirmed
- ☐ I feel good about myself
- ☐ I feel rejuvenated
- ☐ I feel positive
- ☐ I am excited about my future
- ☐ I feel beautiful

- ☐ I am finding out who I am
- ☐ I am rediscovering myself
- ☐ I am angry
- ☐ _____
- ☐ _____
- _____

We hope that you are experiencing some of these life-affirming emotions, even if they only come in short bursts. Many women, in the time immediately following a separation, only experience these more positive emotions in small amounts, and there are many things that may push you back into the grieving part of the healing process.

If you look back at the diagram, you will notice that the bottom part of the loop is labelled Grieving. Women report to us that, as they move through this part of the process, they experience some of the emotions listed below. Check off those that fit for you.

Grieving Emotions

- ☐ I feel that things are hopeless
- ☐ I feel helpless
- ☐ I am afraid for myself
- ☐ I am afraid for my children
- ☐ I worry about the long term impact on my children
- ☐ I regret my children are not having the life I want for them
- ☐ I can't make long-term decisions
- ☐ I feel hurt

- ☐ I feel like I am only enduring life
- ☐ I see no possibilities
- ☐ I am depressed
- ☐ I feel like I am suffocating
- ☐ I feel nauseous
- ☐ I grieve the friends I have lost
- ☐ I worry about losing more friends
- ☐ I grieve the family I have lost (his family too)
- ☐ I worry about money

- [ ] I feel pain
- [ ] I am sad
- [ ] I am lonely
- [ ] I feel like a failure
- [ ] I am frustrated
- [ ] I experience regret
- [ ] I feel guilty
- [ ] I feel shame
- [ ] I am afraid to trust people
- [ ] I feel betrayed by family and friends
- [ ] I feel unsettled and in a constant state of transition
- [ ] I feel confused

- [ ] I grieve what I thought my future was going to look like
- [ ] I fear that I will never have a good relationship with a man
- [ ] I feel anxious
- [ ] I feel like I can't make it on my own
- [ ] I am exhausted
- [ ] I feel overwhelmed
- [ ] I have poor health
- [ ] I am angry
- [ ] _____
    _____
- [ ] _____

For many women, the healing process is a process of 'cycling' through this figure 8 (see diagram on page 98), sometimes feeling and naming all of the losses they have experienced, other times moving forward with their lives. As with most things that have to do with our emotions, it is not all neat and tidy. You may spend hours and even days in the rebuilding part of the process and then, suddenly, find yourself swept back into grief. Similarly, you may be spending a great deal of time in grief, feeling many powerful and uncomfortable emotions and then, without warning, feel great joy or hope at the smallest of things. We have put an opening at the top and bottom of the figure 8, a reminder that some day you will move out of this intense emotional process.

You may also have times when you are in neither part of this figure 8. We spoke earlier about frozen grief, and this may be what is happening for you. Sometimes you may feel so overwhelmed by your situation that you "numb out" from many of your emotions both positive and painful. In the days immediately after leaving her partner, Cate wrote in her journal, "There are so many thoughts in my head. I can't process them all, so I won't process any of them. I am shutting down."

There are all kinds of things that may cause you to "shut down." If you are fearful for your life, fighting in court for your children, or living with a high level of stress you may feel that all you can do is survive.

Once again, be kind to yourself. We believe that there are times when "surviving the day" shows immense courage and determination. Also, it is our experience that once you are out of this intense period of crisis you will have emotional energy for your healing process.

Why am I so angry?

You will notice that anger appears in both of the preceeding lists. How is it that you may be feeling anger in both the rebuilding and grieving phases of the healing process? We believe that anger plays an important role in healing and that there is more than one type of anger. Some anger may feel energizing. It may help you to "stay strong" and "fight" for what is right. It is an anger that propels you forward to build a better life. Many women find that, if they can harness this anger, it can be a powerful fuel for accomplishing the difficult tasks ahead of them.

There is also anger that is more associated with grief. As women add up all of the losses in their lives, they feel angry. They feel they have been robbed. It is very difficult to know what to do with this anger. You are, in fact, angry at your partner and all of the damage he has caused you, but it is not safe to express your anger towards him. You may also feel angry with people or institutions that have let you down, but there is usually little you can do to "right" these "wrongs." Consequently, some women describe the anger as "simmering" inside them. This type of anger tends to be more immobilizing and oppressive, and sometimes women feel paralyzed by it. Other times, women are afraid of the rage they feel building up inside them and worry about what they might be capable of doing. It is important to let yourself experience this very justified anger and find safe places to talk about it. Try writing in a journal or joining a women's support group. These are all important parts of the healing process.

You may also find it hard to feel angry. You may be feeling a new level of anger, some of your feelings and thoughts may be frightening, and many of us have been raised with the message that women should not be angry. Furthermore, your abusive partner demonstrated how harmful anger can be. Remember that anger is not the problem – it is a normal, healthy human emotion. Given all of the ways you have been hurt, it is appropriate to feel angry. The challenge becomes what to do with that anger. As we said before, whenever possible try to use your anger to empower you to take steps towards a better life. When your anger is more disempowering, acknowledge it as part of the healing process, and try to find a helpful way to express it. Anger is not generally pleasant, but you will be glad to know that it doesn't last forever. In our experience, the intense and sometimes frightening level of anger you may be feeling now will subside over time.

Is there something wrong with me?

Healing from the kind of trauma and loss you have experienced is messy. Many women fear that they might be "going crazy." We don't think you are going crazy; in fact, we think you are doing important emotional work no matter what part of the figure 8 you are spending most of your time in.

The intense grief you are experiencing may lead you to see a counselor. Hopefully, that counselor understands your experience and is supportive. However, you may be seeing someone who hasn't made the connection between your complicated grief, all of the impacts of abuse, and your feelings of depression, fear and fatigue. Some counselors or support people might label you with a mental health problem such as depression or anxiety. What is really being named are some of the impacts of abuse. Sometimes a woman does find it helpful to take medication for a while, but it is important to remember you are having a normal human reaction to external circumstances.

Similarly, your physical health may be affected as you work through this intense healing process. Chest pains, stomach problems, headaches and chronic fatigue are all examples of physical ailments that women sometimes experience as they process what has happened to them. While you don't want to ignore these physical symptoms and should have them checked by your doctor, most women find that they subside over time.

Unfortunately, you may find that many people in your life, while able to support you in the rebuilding part of the process, will criticize you for grieving. Many women are accused of not "moving on," and they may even be told that there is something wrong with them. On any given day, in any given moment, whether you are grieving or rebuilding, you are on the journey of healing. Honour yourself for the hard emotional work that you are doing.

I haven't left my partner, so why do I feel like I'm grieving?

Whether or not you have left your partner, you are still facing a great deal of loss and grief. Your relationship is not the way you want it to be. If you have children, they do not have the kind of father you would want for them. It is natural and normal for you to feel sad for all of the things that are not going as you had planned.

Why does the end of a "bad" relationship still hurt so much?

As we have said, sometimes friends, family, neighbours, employers and others do not understand the pain you may be going through. They think you should just be happy to be out of a "bad" relationship. Remember that what you are in the middle of is an immensely complex healing process.

While you are grieving, you may begin to recognize impacts and wounds from your ex-partner's abuse. Meanwhile, the abuse may be ongoing, and there may be new impacts.

It is helpful to remind yourself that in most other situations, when we grieve, it is because of the end of something. Someone has died or we have lost our home or our job. In this case, there is no clear-cut termination. Your partner is not dead; rather he very likely continues to hurt you on an almost daily basis. (This is particularly true if you have children in common.) There is no closure but rather a continual rewounding. It is also very likely that you will remember your partner's "good qualities" after leaving the relationship. After reading this book, you may realize that his apparent kindness and goodness were often a means of manipulating you; it was part of the honeymoon. Still, that goodness felt authentic to you at the time, and, of course, most men who are abusive do have positive qualities. You would never have stayed with him if this were not the case. And so, perhaps you remember the "good times" you had together and feel a longing for what you have lost.

Because the healing process you are moving through is so complex and intense, you are at a particularly vulnerable time in your life. Many women feel like their emotions are scattered all over the place. Both grieving and rebuilding take an enormous amount of emotional energy. We think it is important to be aware of your potential vulnerability. For this reason, we usually caution women against beginning a new relationship while they are still healing. Friends and family may encourage you to "get back out there and date," but trust your instincts and give yourself the time you need to heal from all that you have suffered.

Is it always going to be this painful?

Many women despair at how long the healing process takes. They wonder when they will "be done." First of all, it is helpful to know that this process of rebuilding and grieving does take a long time. Despite your fears, you are not crazy for feeling intense and divergent emotions. You are doing crucial emotional healing work.

Secondly, women tell us over and over again that it does get better. In time you will find your emotions less intense and your mind less consumed by this process. Women who have been free of abuse for some time report having days when they "feel normal" again.

Also, the healing process itself will alter over time. Early on, many women spend the majority of their time in grief. This is natural for anyone experiencing a significant loss. Eventually however, most women tell us that they spend more time rebuilding. After years of being "shut down" by their partner's controlling behaviour, women find great joy in exploring new relationships and experiences. Sometimes women learn new things about themselves. Some women discover gifts and abilities they never knew they had.

If you have been separated for quite a while, you may be spending much of your time in the rebuilding part of the figure 8. However, you will likely find that there are a number of "triggering events" that will pull you back into the grief. Women report to us that sights, smells and memories will trigger grief for them. As well, major events like birthdays, anniversaries and Christmas may stir up feelings of sadness. Events within your extended family may also do this. For example, a wedding or a funeral that puts you in the same room as your ex-partner can be difficult.

There is no right or wrong way to heal from the trauma you have experienced. Some days you will feel overjoyed to be "free" of the relationship. Other days you will feel very sad as you identify yet another thing that you have lost. Be patient with yourself and try to surround yourself with people who understand what a long and complex journey you are on. Finally, be assured that you will get through this. We have had the pleasure of working with hundreds of women over many years. We have been privileged to watch these women grow in new and exciting ways, creating rich and meaningful lives for themselves. You will too!

Can I look forward with hope?

We conclude our book with five stories from women who have found reasons to be hopeful. Their stories help us to see that hope takes different forms in different situations. If not today, then someday soon you too will be able to share a story of hope.

I only left my partner a few months ago, but I already feel much clearer and stronger. I really couldn't see just how bad things were until I got out and had a taste of what it means not to live on edge all of the time. **Gillian**

Living with Brian for 22 years left me a shell of a person. He destroyed my sense of self. I felt unlovable and unacceptable. I doubted everything about myself. Separation and divorce has been hard and is still hard. I've spent a lot of money on lawyers, and I've struggled to help my family and friends understand. But, as hard as it's been, I am so glad that I left when I did. I have slowly come alive as a person. I make my own decisions and have control over my life. One thing I would want to tell other women is "it gets better!" As challenging as my life is, it is so much better than it was before. **Marcia**

I am very thankful that my husband is changing. I know that doesn't happen often. It has taken years for him to rebuild my trust, but now I experience a lot of comfort and security. At the same time, I have worked all along to strengthen myself. Reading this book, finding a great support group, and putting safeguards in place allowed me to stay while he did the work he needed to do. I feel hopeful about our future together, but I am also certain beyond a doubt that I will never go back to the way we once were. I hope our marriage will survive and grow stronger and stronger, but at the same time I know now that I will be okay whatever happens. **Sylvia**

I left Sean three years ago, and I am now in a loving and respectful relationship with a new person. He is so completely different from my first partner. I never really realized what I was missing out on until I got it. Glen always keeps my best interests in mind. He accepts me and appreciates me for who I am. We are best friends. We can talk about anything. He is real, faithful, and honest, and he treats me like an equal. My spirit feels at peace when I am with him. **Julie**

I regret ever meeting Larry, but I sure don't regret leaving him. As painful and hard as all of this has been, I am glad I am finally "out." I feel like I have myself back. Once again, I know who I am. I feel strong. I can dream my own dreams and think my own thoughts. I feel like I have a future with hope. **Carol**

Afterword

For many years women have shared their stories with us. In turn, in the pages of this book, we have shared their stories with you. We truly appreciate the gift they have given us. Each woman's story is a treasure—a witness to her strength, courage and wisdom. We have used parts of their stories throughout our book because the truth about violence against women lies in the stories of the women themselves. For us, abuse against women is not a theory or a social phenomenon; it is what happens to real women. Although each woman's story is unique, there are remarkable similarities in the experiences, thoughts and feelings of women when the person they love abuses them. They wrestle with the same dilemmas and confusions.

We hope that what you have read in this book has reassured you that you are truly not alone. There are others who can understand and appreciate the overwhelming situation in which you find yourself.

We also hope that this book has helped you to begin to trust your own story and to honour your own strength, courage and wisdom.

Order more copies of

When Love Hurts

A Woman's Guide to Understanding
Abuse in Relationships

*Jill Cory &
Karen McAndless-Davis*

Second Edition

Cost $19.95

www.whenlovehurts.ca | info@whenlovehurts.ca

Please inquire about discounts for bulk orders.

The Authors of

When Love Hurts

A Woman's Guide to Understanding Abuse in Relationships

Second Edition

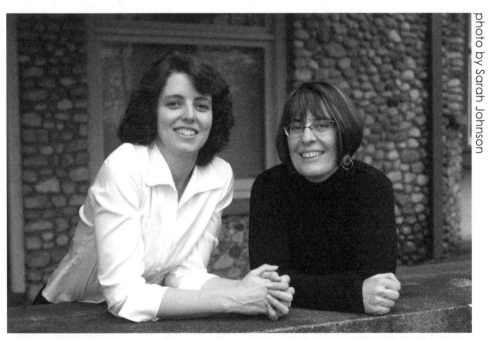

Karen McAndless-Davis (on the left) and Jill Cory (on the right)

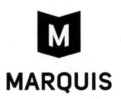

MARQUIS

Québec, Canada

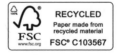

RECYCLED
Paper made from
recycled material
FSC® C103567

Printed on Enviro 100% post-consumer EcoLogo certified paper,
processed chlorine free and manufactured using biogas energy.

    BIO GAS